Speech Pathology and Audiology:
Iowa Origins of a Discipline

Speech Pathology
&
Audiology

Iowa Origins of a Discipline

Dorothy Moeller

The University of Iowa   Iowa City
1975

Library of Congress Cataloging in Publication Data

Moeller, Dorothy.
  Speech pathology & audiology.

  Includes bibliographies and index.
    1. Speech, Disorders of—Study and teaching—Iowa—
History. 2. Audiology—Study and teaching—Iowa—
History. 3. Iowa. University. I. Title.
RC428.M63   616.8'55'0711777655   75-45237
ISBN 0-87745-066-8

CONTENTS

Introduction   *ix*

1   Beginnings of Beginnings   1

2   Psychologist of Psychiatry   14

3   The Travis Period: *NRC, 1924-1927*   25

4   The Travis Period: *People and Climate*   39

5   The Travis Period: *1927-1938*   58

6   The Strother Period: *1939-1947*   86

7   The Johnson Period: *1947-1955*   113

8   The Curtis Period: *1955-1968*   154

Index (Proper names, organizations, journals)   209

Index (Subject)   215

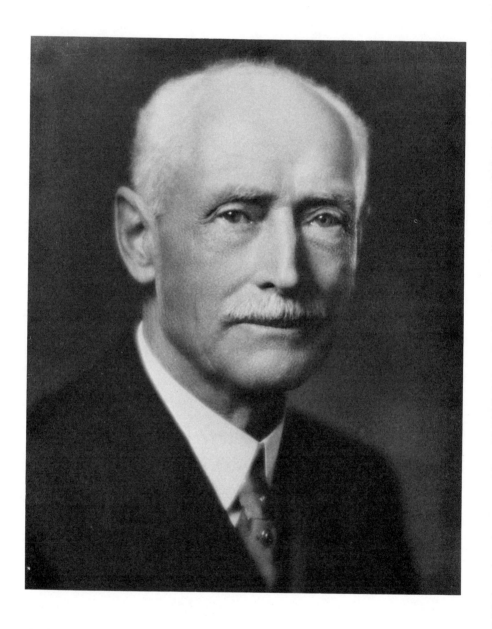

Carl Emil Seashore

1866-1949

To Carl Emil Seashore,
with deep respect,
and in gratitude
for those splendid contributions
to The University of Iowa
that flowered in the Iowa origins
of a new discipline, today called
speech pathology and audiology.

INTRODUCTION

The University of Iowa's Department of Speech Pathology and Audiology sponsored the research and writing of this history of Iowa origins of the discipline of speech pathology and audiology and of Iowa contributions to the development of that discipline within the University and nationally. The period chosen is from 1883 to 1968, that is, from beginnings of beginnings to the dedication of the department's new home, the Wendell Johnson Speech and Hearing Center.

Dr. James F. Curtis, Department Chairman, initiated the project, guided it through its formative stages, and with his colleagues gave counsel on the evolving statement. His successor, Dr. Kenneth L. Moll, was concerned primarily with the final draft and with arrangements for publication.

There were two purposes. The first was to provide a well-documented and dependable text for use as a reference tool. The second was to sketch in the background in order to present the remarkable human side of the story of scholarly and disciplined venturing in the laboratory, the classroom, and the clinic: a story that had become a legend in its own time but had never been put to paper except in bits and pieces.

By joining these purposes, the history stands replete with incident and with names, idea, and innovations of early day giants of the University: Dr. Patrick, Dean Seashore, President Jessup, Dr. Orton, Prof. Mabie, Dr. Dean, Dr. Stewart. And it follows, generation by generation, the successes—and failures—of those who came later but who, like Seashore and the others, have tried to discover new knowledges, new understandings, and new procedures helpful in handling those frustrating personal problems that center in impairment of speech or hearing or both. The statement, therefore, reaches beyond the profession and the world of academe to touch the human community.

The text is drawn from personal interviews, correspondence, conversations, and the fragmentary but considerable documentary evidence to be found in journal articles, monographs, and books by or concerning persons or activities that have a place in the story. Writings of Seashore, Johnson, and Patrick have proven of great value.

Many individuals have been involved throughout the project. Seventeen gave taped interviews: Dr. Lee Edward Travis of Los Angeles; Dr. Margaret Hall Powers of Chicago; Dr. Charles Strother of Seattle; Dr. Ernest Henrickson and Dr. Bryng Bryngelson of Minneapolis; and twelve present or former members of The University of Iowa faculty, in Iowa City. The twelve were Dr. Curtis, Dr. Jay Melrose, Dr. Dorothy Sherman, Bette Spriestersbach, Dr. D. C. Spriestersbach, and Dr. Dean Williams, Speech Pathology and Audiology; Dr. Don Lewis and Prof. Ted Hunter, Psychology; Dr. John Knott, Psychiatry; Dr. Dean Lierle, Dr. Scott Reger, and Prof. Jeanne Smith, Otolaryngology and Maxillofacial Surgery.

These seventeen also read and critically appraised the manuscript as did three others of the University faculty: Dr. Spencer Brown, who had returned to Iowa for a time with an appointment in the Department of Pediatrics, Dr. Moll and Dr. Hughlett Morris, Speech Pathology and Audiology. Dr. Paul Huston, Psychiatry, made available documents from archives in his department. Bessie Rasmus Petersen, earlier of the Department of Speech, shared recollections of the Orton-Travis period.

Many, on request, gave information through correspondence. Among these were Dr. John Black, Dr. Brown, Dr. Milton Cowan, Dr. Frederic L. Darley, Lois Cobb Kluver, Mrs. E. C. Mabie, Dr. Milton Metfessel, Mrs. Earl Schubert, Dr. Hildred Schuell, Florence Teager, Dr. William Tiffany, Dr. Joseph Tiffin, Dr. Charles Van Riper, and Betty Walker. Ms. Walker also made a gift of her cherished scrapbook of newspaper clippings of the Travis period. This scrapbook, the interview tapes, and other materials collected in the research have been placed in the archives of the Department of Speech Pathology and Audiology.

Several members of the University faculty and staff gave service in locating information, among them Ann Evans, Psychology-Education Library; Robert Hedges, University Archives; Winifred Tanberg, Psychology office; Margaret Seemuth and Varena Wade, Speech Pathology and Audiology office; and Lillian Yeggy, Personnel office. Ms. Wade also typed the several versions of the manuscript.

The project was supported partially by funds from the Department of Speech Pathology and Audiology, the Graduate College of the University, and the Louis W. and Maud Hill Family Foundation of St. Paul. Publication was made possible by the generous financial aid of alumni and friends and by the interest and assistance of the University of Iowa Foundation.

The author acknowledges with pleasure her indebtedness to those named, and to the many not named but warmly remembered, for wise advice and kind encouragement. She, of course, takes responsibility for errors, infelicities, or inadvertencies that may have found their way into the text in spite of much checking and in spite of the friendly watchfulness of the staff of the Department of Publications and of Janet Whitebook of the Department of Speech Pathology and Audiology, who served as liaison between the department and the Press.

Because history seems limited essentially to what is remembered and recorded, and because in that imperfect situation much is overlooked, she suggests a salute to the hundreds of teachers and students and clients who happened not to have been so recorded but who were on hand, joining in the venturing as they could and adding thus to the richness of the legacy celebrated in these pages.

—D. M.

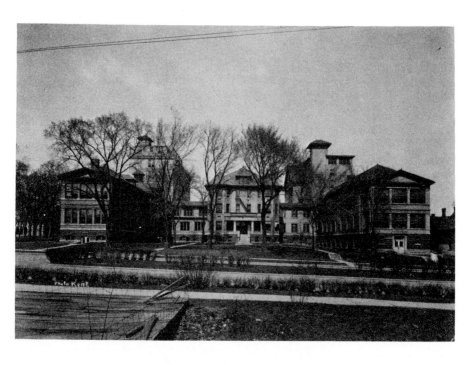

The original home of the Department of Speech Pathology and Audiology, East Hall, as it appeared when it was still University Hospital (circa 1924).

1

BEGINNINGS OF BEGINNINGS

Beginnings of beginnings of speech pathology at The University of Iowa go back at least as far as the graduate student days of one George Thomas White Patrick, and the academic turmoil of about a century ago when he and others like him helped to move the study of human behavior out of the armchair and into the laboratory. He was one of the young scholars who broke away from the book-and-lecture approach of the venerable discipline of philosophy to become part of an innovative movement which many regarded as brash and undignified, and which came to be called the new psychology. It was laboratory-centered. It borrowed its methodology from science. And its fundamental proposition was that the study of man is the study of man. (The history recorded in these pages carries the story of the development of that proposition at Iowa, in matters related to problems of speech and hearing, through the next eight and a half decades, that is, through the period that ends in 1968 with the dedication of the Wendell Johnson Speech and Hearing Center.)

G. T. W. Patrick was a soft spoken, frail looking gentleman from Vermont who earned his B.A. degree at The University of Iowa in 1878, and who nine years later joined the Iowa faculty as professor and head of Mental and Moral Science and Didactics. That nine year period was memorable. He began his studies at Yale. Then he had continued them at Johns Hopkins, with G. Stanley Hall, in the only psychological laboratory in the United States (opened in 1883), and under Hall's direction had all but completed his doctorate—he was granted leave in May 1888 to do this. And, finally, he had worked with Wilhelm Wundt, in Wundt's famous laboratory in Leipzig, the first (1879) psychological laboratory in the world.

Years later, in an autobiographical sketch (6), Patrick compressed this great experience into a masterful understatement: "Some of this I brought to Iowa." By "this" he meant the vision and the spirit and the techniques of the new psychology as he had been introduced to them by Wundt, generally considered the father of the new science, and by Hall, one of Wundt's first students and a first generation man in the science in this country.

In 1887 there was no professorship in psychology in the United States or Europe, and there were few course titles using the word. But that year Patrick offered a course at The University of Iowa called Empirical

Psychology. What is more, in this course he used some tuning forks and brain models and charts, as he had seen Hall and Wundt use them. This was the beginning of the Iowa Psychological Laboratory which continues to this day, and which has been listed in the University catalogue ever since 1890. If 1887 is taken as the founding date, the Iowa laboratory and one opened that fall at Pennsylvania by Cattell share honors in this country as next after Hall's; if 1890 is taken as the date, the Iowa laboratory is fourth or fifth in the nation—a pioneer either way.

Patrick spent all of his expense money that first year, a total of $50, to buy his laboratory equipment, and in explaining *(7)* this squandering of resources wrote the administration that when he came to Iowa he "had in mind no other plan than to have a psychological laboratory both for demonstration and research." From then on his budget included money for laboratory equipment, but for some years everything that was owned could be kept in the "cabinet with the glass doors." He dissected a sheep's brain at the first meeting of this class in 1888, a fact which becomes of more than passing interest in view of the pioneering work Lee Travis was to do with brain waves early in the Iowa Program.

Patrick brought to Iowa not only the culture of the new psychology but also, in 1897, a man named Seashore—Carl Emil Seashore—to be director of the Iowa Psychological Laboratory and Professor of Philosophy. Seashore shared Patrick's enormous enthusiasm for the new psychology and had perhaps an even greater enthusiasm for instrumentation.

SEASHORE AND THE NEW PSYCHOLOGY

Seashore had been a graduate student at Yale, studying with George Trumbull Ladd, when, in 1892, Ladd invited E. W. Scripture, "who had come out of the psychological laboratory at Leipzig," to open a laboratory as an instructor in psychology. "Naturally," wrote Seashore (*10*, pp. 11, 12) many years later,

> I registered for this new course. It soon became apparent that he did not show what I thought was decent respect for the psychology of Ladd and his associates. Though thoroughly courteous, he took the position that psychology has to start from scratch. He conveyed the impression that the systematic statements in the learned books of the day might all be true, but they were nevertheless second-hand. This difference was very difficult for me to grasp, because I had the highest admiration for the wonderful acumen and power of exposition I was finding in Ladd and his associates. . . . It seemed to me that Scripture had nothing to say or demonstrate that was in any respect comparable to Ladd's massive array of psychological facts.
>
> The issue, however, came to a crisis in the selection of my topic for

the doctoral dissertation. Going to Ladd, I said, 'I would like to perform some experiments on the power of inhibition,' a topic on which I then had only an inceptive but rather enticing notion. He said, 'Yes, Mr. Seashore, that is a very interesting topic. You will find a fairly full account of it in my large volume, *Elements of Psychology*.' ... I found the statement very lucid and comprehensive, and that put a damper on my enthusiasm for experimentation.

Not being entirely at ease, I went across Elm Street to Scripture and said, 'I am very much interested in the subject of inhibition and would like to see if I can perform some experiments on that subject.' Scripture, being an exceedingly formal and dignified person, for the first time eliminated the 'Mr.' and, slapping me on the shoulder, said, 'Good, Seashore, try it.' This had a magnetic effect; although then ignorant of what it implied, I date the birth of my scientific attitude from that moment. For the first time I sensed a feeling of companionship in a creative approach to psychology and felt that the laboratory was going to give me satisfaction which could well compare with the deep satisfaction I had felt in the learned and all-comprehensive textbooks.

Half a century later, Seashore began an article on "Applied Psychology in 1895" with these three words: "There wasn't any!" He called the new psychology almost a "science on faith," because there was so little to work with in terms of either information or instrumentation. There were

but few of the tools of investigation. Psychological instruments were waiting for invention and marketing, and physics offered but little help at the time. . . .

Audiometry had a slow and discouraging rise for twenty-five years. Very few people felt the need of it and those who did had no adequate instruments. . . .

For the first twenty-five years after 1895 very little progress was made in speech pathology. It had no academic status in either psychology or medicine. Scripture launched the treatment of stuttering through the publication of his book on that subject but, as he went abroad to live in England and Switzerland at that time, there was no significant follow-up for several years. The treatment of stuttering was in the hands of private individuals and sporadic institutions of more or less doubtful standing. The thing that justified academic recognition for speech pathology was the development of graduate work in the psychology of speech and the admission of clinical psychology into psychopathic hospitals. This justified the establishment of speech clinics.

PATRICK AND SEASHORE

Though Patrick was a Vermonter and Seashore was born in Sweden, the two men had much in common. Both had grown up on Iowa farms, both had known the rigors of pioneer life.

Patrick, as an undergraduate at Iowa, had lived in a room heated by a wood stove for which he split and carried fuel upstairs daily all winter. He and a friend once toted a trunk the mile from Myrtle Avenue to the Rock Island depot to save a quarter. He kept books for a Colorado mine for three years after he received his Iowa B.A. to finance his graduate work at Yale, and with Hall and Wundt.

Seashore's family had come from Sweden to Boone County when he was three. "Resistance to the cold, struggle against the elements in every way was," he once wrote *(9),* "an opportunity for overcoming difficulties and feeling success. This kept our blood red and our muscles firm and our appetites good." But in addition to similar backgrounds—and perhaps this was even more important—Patrick and Seashore shared the experience of having studied with first generation people of the new psychology, and of having found excitement and challenge and satisfaction in this new science.

Their working relationship appears to have been pleasant and productive from the first. The new man did not have to do battle with the old for the new way of thinking and the new way of doing things—instead he received warm support and every encouragement.

When Seashore arrived on the Iowa campus in 1897 he spent his first summer supervising the building of the soundproof room in the department's new quarters in the Liberal Arts building (now Schaeffer Hall); as far as he knew this was the only sound-, light-, and jar-proof room of its kind in existence at that time. It was built *(10,* pp. 28, 29; *7)* "on the principle of a gigantic thermos bottle standing on a towering support of sand piers." That fall he continued his basic research in music, voice, and hearing, and with the building of instruments, including audiometers and tonoscopes, often working from plans he and Scripture had talked about or experimented with at Yale. For the next four years he practically lived in the Psychological Laboratory—the workshop as he called it. He was (10, p. 9) his own "mechanician, secretary, textbook writer, instrument builder, and general flunky in charge of the rooms of the department including the library."

SEASHORE'S AUDIOMETER AND EXPERIMENTATION

In 1900 Seashore had brought the development of his audiometer to the point at which it was taken over by Stoelting, and for about fifteen years it was the only audiometer on the market except Scripture's original model, which Seashore had helped build when he was at Yale. Stoelting sold many Seashore audiometers but Seashore *(10,* pp. 39-43), "to encourage his [Stoelting's] pioneering in the building of psychological instruments . . .

refused to accept any royalty either for this or other instruments" of his marketed by Stoelting. "Being a scientific instrument, it [the audiometer] was not patented."

Describing the building of his audiometer Seashore continued,

> The first problem I tackled after coming to Iowa was that of designing an audiometer suitable for use both in the laboratory and in the schools. After considerable experimenting I built this first audiometer with my own hands. It was long after this that the term 'decibel' was coined, but it was interesting that in this rule-of-thumb procedure I had hit upon the approximate present decibel magnitude as a unit in forty steps and had made it linear through the choice of a fitting logarithmic scale of intensities.

In those early years Seashore also did a considerable amount of research in psychoacoustics. He designed a wide range of experiments and instrumentation in a continuing effort to discover ways of identifying and measuring dimensions of sound.

His work at this point was enhanced by a change in the administrative framework. In 1900 the Program in Mental and Moral Science and Didactics had become the Department of Philosophy and Psychology, with Patrick continuing as head. In 1905 Seashore succeeded Patrick in this position; with that change Seashore became also the central figure in the pioneering efforts out of which the Iowa Program in Speech Pathology would develop. Patrick remained on the faculty until 1926, but did most of his later work in philosophy. The department was divided in 1927 into separate departments of Philosophy and Psychology, with Seashore as head of the latter.

In 1908 Seashore became Dean of the Graduate College, and continued as department head, and in this expanded role proceeded to use his commitment to the laboratory approach, his genius for leadership, and the power of his position to initiate and support new programs throughout the entire University. As one of his biographers (5) has put it, "The University gave him great scope and he used it with grace and skill." Another (3) is more specific, suggesting that "fortunately" Seashore took advantage of his dual administrative positions "to promote his own personal academic interests" and that among these were "the psychology of music, the psychology of reading disability, the Child Welfare Research Station, the School of Religion, the Psychopathic Hospital, student placement examinations, speech pathology and what he called the 'psychology of otology.' The psychology of otology today is included within the framework of audiology." His influence in applied psychology in relation to the professions and higher education was to become worldwide.

SEASHORE'S COMMITMENT TO RESEARCH

Seashore's fundamental commitment was to basic research. As he once explained (*10*, p. 24), there are two approaches to applied psychology. One is for the psychologist to go out and render a service with the material in hand. The other is "to introduce some sound psychological technique for laying a cornerstone to a possible structure in some field of applied psychology." He chose the latter approach, but with a strong feeling for the human uses of the techniques and understandings which the laboratory might yield. And so he gave himself, also, to the development of certain clinical programs when he estimated that scientific research had established an adequate foundation for them. His central idea of the purpose of education (*5*) was to keep all students busy at their highest natural level of successful achievement. He was "interested in everything, and if it were possible for him to help, he wanted to help—and he did help."

It was perhaps his laboratory orientation for collecting all available data to bear on a problem that led him to draw people from various disciplines to work in a common purpose. It was said of him (*2*, pp. 4,5) that he seemed to

> promote interdepartmentalism by means of nearly every major administrative decision he made. It was one of his basic convictions that the most significant discoveries and developments were to be come upon in what he called the borderline regions of the academic and scientific world, and that the exploration and cultivation of these borderline areas required the crossing over of departmental lines, the relaxing of departmental sovereignties in certain respects, and the cooperation of all those whose territory was jointly affected. . . . [He was an] unresting organizer of teams . . . and it was a curious and provocative fact that every time Dean Seashore destroyed or gravely damaged a departmental barrier he tended to bring into being a new kind of specialist—a person peculiarly trained to serve as captain for a new kind of team made up of old kinds of specialists with a new sense of purpose.

In this "bold expansion into applied fields" (*10*, p. 11) the work in four areas, in addition to psychology as such, was to relate meaningfully to the institution's readiness for the Program in Speech Pathology. These areas were mental hygiene, child development, otology, and speech, with speech ranking first in importance after psychology.

Mental Hygiene. "At the beginning of this [the twentieth] century the term 'mental hygiene' had not come into general use nor had preventive medicine gained any distinctive recognition," Seashore (*10*, pp. 122-159) explained. There was no psychiatrist in Iowa. Clinical psychology was not known here—or anywhere, for that matter, for that discipline did not appear as such in the academic world until the forties. There was one small sanitarium in the state, and the heads of insane asylums—that's what they were called—were primarily business managers. So, to fill a felt need, in 1908 Seashore established the Iowa Psychological Clinic at The University of Iowa for cases of mental pathology, organizing the clinic around coursework in abnormal psychology. "This innovation in American psychology was recognized," he wrote (*10*, p. 124). "It was significant that I was invited to be a guest of Clark University at the invitation of G. Stanley Hall [Patrick's mentor who had left Johns Hopkins to become president of Clark] for a week's series of lectures and conferences by Freud, Jung, and E. E. Jones."

Seashore proceeded to work not only within the University but also throughout the state to develop interest in a mental health program. His hope was that an experimental hospital could be established as a clearing-house for mental patients and that his Psychological Clinic of Mental Pathology could be integrated with an outpatient clinic for children.

He and colleagues at the University finally developed a legislative program aimed at achieving these goals. Working with him on this was a typically interdisciplinary committee composed of Dr. E. F. Van Epps, a clinical neurologist, Professor B. G. Bolton, from the Department of Education, Dean M. B. Guthrie, of the College of Medicine, and University President George E. MacLean. The legislation was passed in 1919, establishing the Psychopathic Hospital as a teaching, research, and training facility at the University, with the Psychological Clinic of Mental Pathology as an integral part. Dr. Samuel T. Orton became the first director of the hospital and program.

Child Development. During the years he was involved with the mental health campaign, Seashore became active in another project which had been proceeding with difficulty for almost a decade. A number of Iowa citizens had been working that long for some kind of state-supported enterprise for the study of the well child. No such project was known in the state, or anywhere else for that matter. But to those working for it, the lack in Iowa seemed particularly unfortunate because here there was a flourishing program for the study of farm animals. "All that money for hogs and cattle and not a cent for children," they used to say. They went to the legislature several times, but with no success.

Then they asked Seashore for help. And he gave it: he joined them and their cause. In 1917 the legislature established in Iowa, as an adjunct of the University, the Iowa Child Welfare Research Station (known since 1963 as the Institute of Child Behavior and Development). This was the first such facility in the world, that is, the first to be concerned scientifically and systematically with the behavior and development of the well, normal child.

Dr. Bird T. Baldwin became the director of the Station where the program was activated very soon after the legislative decision of 1917. Graduate students who began to work in the area were drawn from various disciplines, including many from psychology and speech, since children's speech was one of the first behaviors chosen for study. An M.A. thesis completed there in 1919 by Sara Stinchfield (Hawk), a psychology major who went on to have a distinguished career in speech pathology, was concerned with children's speech problems including stuttering. This reference to stuttering was apparently the first in a thesis at The University of Iowa, and is one of the very earliest in the literature, since in those years the scientific inquiry into speech problems was all but unknown. The Stinchfield thesis included tests for teachers to use in assessing the adequacy of a pupil's speech.

Otology. Seashore's fundamental research in sound had led him to studies of vocalization, and this in turn had interested him in the psychological aspects of the production of vocal sounds by humans. This interest produced a cooperative arrangement with the Department of Otology and Ophthalmology[1] in the College of Medicine, in particular with Dr. L. W. Dean, the head of that department. The two men came to work together often on doctoral committees; the relationship between their two departments remained close through the years and would come to contribute significantly to the Iowa Program in Speech Pathology.

One of the landmark interdisciplinary doctoral programs drawn up and directed by Seashore and Dr. Dean involved the training of C. C. Bunch, a graduate student in psychology who had worked with both of them in developing the Iowa Pitch Range Audiometer *(3)*, and whose further training, at the doctoral level, involved work on the practical application of methods of testing hearing. This was an area of first interest to Seashore who carried on a very long one-man campaign with educators and the medical profession for recognition of the need for improved methods of testing hearing.

The Iowa Pitch Range Audiometer played an important part in this project. This audiometer turned out to be Seashore's final one for the pleasant reason that the Bell Telephone Company, after considerable urging from him, finally took interest in the hearing testing problem and went into it as a large-scale scientific investigation. "It is significant to note," Seashore added *(10,* p. 40), "that this was at the beginning of the policy of this great institution . . . to go extensively into pure research." In recognition of Seashore's work the company gave the University one of its first 1-A audiometers, an instrument it developed early in its new program.

After Bunch received the Ph.D. degree in 1920, Seashore referred to him as a psychologist of otology. The so-called psychology of otology, which grew in Dr. Dean's department, first under Bunch and then under others, would eventually be included in modern day audiology.

Speech. Since the turn of the century, the University had had a Chair in Public Speaking in the English Department for instruction in elocution and in what was generally referred to as artistic speech, that is, general speech with a tinge of the dramatic. Seashore *(1)* saw possibilities for psychological research here, and wished to have someone on the staff who could "exploit the area of the speech arts." So in 1912 Glenn Merry, a graduate student in psychology who had a certificate from the Cumnock School of Oratory (later Northwestern University's School of Speech), was named to head this Public Speaking unit. The appointment was made by Clark Ansley, head of the English Department. Merry proceeded to read and to travel, as well as to study in many departments of the University to prepare for the new program. According to Seashore,

> He set out to find out all he could about new approaches to the field of speech. He went to Harvard and Columbia. He consulted G. W. Stewart in the Iowa physics department for help in acoustical analysis of speech. He was looking for exact methods by which he could define speech sounds. He . . . studied the research in the psychology of music. He went to the Kay School in Cleveland which was . . . using techniques Merry thought might be applicable to the production of speech. He went into the medical laboratory . . . to study anatomy. And from the studies in physics, anatomy, and psychology he began to learn what it was that made a vocal tone. Merry experimented with x-rays and wrote articles for speech journals on resonance. . . . All of this was to find more objective information on the nature of speech in an attempt to establish a voice science which could contribute objective information about the nature . . . of speech.

SPEECH SCIENCE

To study speech scientifically was a radical change from the old approach, and under Merry's leadership Iowa became the first institution of higher education in the country to recognize, in a department title, "Speech" as opposed to "Public Speaking." Changes in the organization of the academic unit suggest something of the evolution of Merry's program. In 1914 the Chair of Public Speaking in English became the Department of Public Speaking and, in 1921, the Department of Speech. Merry headed each in succession. (This department will be referred to here as the Department of Speech or the Speech Department, even though its full official title is the Department of Speech and Dramatic Art.)

Seashore's new and specific interest in speech and speech problems has been viewed as a logical outgrowth of his earlier interest, the psychology of music, which was itself part of his wide-ranging interest in sound, voice, voice recording, voice tests, musical talent tests, and hearing. Lee Travis, who was to become the first head of the Iowa Program, has seen the development in that way. He *(11)*feels that Seashore

> went very easily over into speech. Remember his famous studies in the vibrato. Here was a voice wave. And this was in speech too. He used to tell us in our classes with him that if you could completely analyze the voice wave you would have a perfect picture of everything you want to know about a human being. I am not sure, any more, that the voice is sufficiently complicated to carry the whole person. But maybe it is, if you could analyze every little harmonic and know what that little harmonic meant in terms of structure and function. But that is what he used to claim, that the whole nature of the person, the true significance of the person, is all in that physical record of the voice.

Seashore is said *(1)*to have felt that at Iowa "the pattern began to change from the old elocution" to the new voice science by 1916. It was in that year that Merry offered two courses which appear to be directly related to beginnings of both laboratory and clinical work in the soon-to-emerge Program in Speech Pathology. One of these courses was "phonology and voice laboratory," and its second-semester continuation, "phonetics and voice laboratory." The other was "voice."

The former, according to the catalogue description, was concerned with "the anatomical and physiological basis of voice, voice analysis, study of voice defects and their removal." Student voices were recorded "for purposes of study." Students possessing "voice defects which are not organic" were urged to register for the course. In the "voice" course there was "intensive study of the voice, special attention being directed toward the remedying of voice defects that are not organic . . . [and toward] the physiological basis of voice production—methods of breathing, resonating, and articulating." The catalogue notation includes a statement about voices being analyzed and "defects" classified.

Merry took a leave of absence for the 1920-21 academic year to complete his own Ph.D. program in psychology. This thesis was on voice inflection in speech. In his acknowledgements he mentions both Seashore and Mabel Claire Williams, also of the Department of Psychology, but no person outside of that department. Apparently the interdisciplinary feature here was of psychology and speech. Merry did most of his research in the Psychological Laboratory about which he wrote this note for the spring 1921 *(4)*issue of the *Quarterly Journal of Speech Education:*

> There is . . . special emphasis at the University of Iowa this year upon the development of an apparatus which now is operating

successfully that will give graphic representation of speech sounds. The voice is first recorded on a phonograph, then reproduced from a record, by means of the apparatus, by a tracing upon a smoked drum. The pitch and intensity values, the rate of utterances and the time values of enunciation of such tracings are easily read and offer an absolute and reproducible bit of evidence as to what occurs in speech so far as sounds are concerned. The apparatus times these elements to within a thousandth of a second which is sufficient for present studies. With this machine it is hoped to make a functional interpretation of the use of pitch emphasis, and other studies in the near future that depend upon an exact and objective method of getting a record of the voice. In this connection studies are being carried on in the psychology of speech.

An earlier note *(12)* in the *Journal* had described briefly other phases of this research.

During his leave of absence for his doctorate he served as chairman of the research committee of the National Association of Teachers of Speech, and in that role began to be known on the national level as a leader in the new scientific approach to the study of speech. His report to the 1920 convention *(4)*, covering a national survey made by his committee, indicated that at that time little graduate work of a strictly research nature was being carried on by departments of speech (or public speaking), and that an M.A. program was then offered at only five institutions: Cornell University, The University of Iowa, the University of Michigan, Valparaiso University, and the University of Wisconsin. "The University of Iowa and Wisconsin are offering this year [1920] work for a minor toward the Ph.D. degree with the probability of offering work for a major toward the Ph.D. degree next year."

Fundamentals Course. Some kind of fundamentals course ("fundamentals" was often used in the title) in public speaking—later speech—had been offered at the University since 1900, and for many years was required of all department majors. Beginning in 1919, and continuing into the fifties when it became part of the so-called communication skills program, this course was required also of all first year liberal arts students. These students became a population from which subjects were drawn for various studies in speech and hearing, and their speech and hearing problems also made evident the need for clinical services.

Foreshadowing of the Clinic. To handle the enlarged enrollment, Merry set up a sizeable staff which came to include, over the years, many students who went on to become speech pathologists. Among them was Miss Arminda Mowre (Iowa B.A. 1922) who had come to Iowa from Montana and who had known Merry when both were at the Cumnock School of Oratory. Early in the new enlarged fundamentals project Merry asked her if she would try to do something for the stutterers who were being found. She said she would. And it was thus, though very informally and on a small scale, that certain clinical work in speech problems got under way.

Seashore, meanwhile, was working toward a speech clinic at the administrative level and in a framework of interdisciplinary action. He had brought together Merry, Dr. Orton, and Dr. Dean, to form what he called the Committee on the Speech Clinic. On July 1, 1921, this committee, according to a letter in the Seashore papers in the University archives, unanimously voted to make these recommendations to President Walter A. Jessup:

that a speech clinic be established;

that the direction be vested "in the present committee";

that the clinic be "so organized as to conserve the chief interests of the Departments of Psychiatry, Speech, Laryngology, and Psychology, as the chief contributors of scientific work in this field";

"that *an effort be made at once to secure the best available specialists for this work* [italics ours]";

and that a sum not to exceed $8,000 be set aside for this appropriation for the first year.

Then the letter, which is signed by Seashore as chairman, ends with this paragraph: "It is unnecessary for me to present a brief for this recommendation as you are thoroughly conversant with the situation— the needs of such a clinic and the very great difficulty of organizing it effectively."

Those recommendations led directly into developments which would integrate certain elements of the new work in psychiatry, child behavior and development, otology, speech, and particularly psychology. Out of that integration would come eventually the Iowa Program in Speech Pathology.

Much of the basic work, then and in years following, was being done by graduate students who were being attracted by the pioneering interdisciplinary programs devised by Seashore and his colleagues. Seashore felt (*10*, p. 115) that this new concept in graduate training was indeed "the key to the rapid development of research for graduate work in formative fields. It drew to the University large numbers of selected and advanced graduate and postdoctorate students who carried the brunt of the burden of research as apprentices."

And so at this point in the beginnings of the Iowa Program, the new psychology could be said to be very much alive on the Iowa campus. Patrick's work, and Hall's, and Wundt's, and Scripture's was going forward dramatically as the stately Seashore strode from one new project to another, crossing department lines almost at will, bringing to the University an era of innovation unprecedented in its history.

REFERENCES

1. Paul Wilson Davee, "Definition of the Philosophy Underlying the Recognition and Teaching of Theater as a Fine Art in the Liberal Arts and Graduate Curricula at the State University of Iowa," Ph.D. dissertation, The University of Iowa, 1950.

2. Wendell Johnson (Ed.), *Stuttering in Children and Adults* (Minneapolis: University of Minnesota Press, 1955).

3. Dean Lierle, with Scott Reger, "The Origin and Development of Audiometric Audiology at the University of Iowa," *Transactions of the American Otological Society, 54,* 1966, 19-23.

4. Glenn Newton Merry and others, "Research in Speech Education," *Quarterly Journal of Speech Education* (now *Quarterly Journal of Speech*), *7,* April 1921, 97-108.

5. Walter R. Miles, "Carl Emil Seashore," in *Biographical Memoirs* (New York: Columbia University Press, 1956, for the National Academy of Sciences of the United States of America), 265-316.

6. G.T.W. Patrick, *Centennial Memoirs,* volume 1, section 2 (Iowa City: University of Iowa Press, 1947), including portions of Patrick's "Founding of the Psychological Laboratory at the State University of Iowa," *Iowa Journal of History and Politics,* July 1932.

7. G.T.W. Patrick, "The New Psychological Laboratory at the University of Iowa," *University of Iowa Studies in Psychology, 3,* 1902, 140-144.

8. Carl Emil Seashore, "Applied Psychology in 1895," *Journal of Speech Disorders, 10,* September 1945, 211-213.

9. Carl Emil Seashore, in Carl Murchison (Ed.), *A History of Psychology in Autobiography* (Worcester: Clark University Press, 1930), volume I, 225-297.

10. Carl Emil Seashore, *Pioneering in Psychology* (Iowa City: University of Iowa Press, 1942).

11. Lee Edward Travis, taped conversation with author, Los Angeles, February 8, 1968.

12. "Voice Inflection in Speech" (author unidentified but probably Merry since this title is also the title of his thesis) in "Notes from the Classroom and Laboratory," *Quarterly Journal of Speech Education* (now *Quarterly Journal of Speech*), *7,* November 1921, 397-8.

NOTE

[1] This department name was changed later to Otolaryngology and Oral Surgery, and since 1952 has been Otolaryngology and Maxillofacial Surgery. Sometimes Seashore called it Laryngology, sometimes Otology.

2

PSYCHOLOGIST OF PSYCHIATRY

"A particular incident gave a significant turn of events at the beginning of the cooperation between psychiatry and psychology," Dean Seashore wrote (*9*, p. 134), under the heading of *Speech Pathology* in a chapter entitled "Clinical Psychology and Psychiatry" in his book, *Pioneering in Psychology*. He continues,

> The case of a child who had a serious reading and speech disability came to the attention of Dr. Orton and he tried what seemed to be a fundamental theory for the interpretation and treatment of such cases.
>
> At that time problems of reading disabilities and speech pathology were in primitive stages. Dr. Orton thought it might be wise to secure as a psychologist a person who was well trained for the development of that unexplored field. A careful survey of the country showed no such person available.
>
> We therefore decided that psychiatry and psychology should undertake the training of a specialist for this field and accordingly selected the most promising senior, encouraging him to go into training for this position. We selected Lee Edward Travis and planned a very comprehensive course of training in psychiatry and psychology for him, the main objective being for specialization in this field.

It was thus that Travis became (*4*, p. 7), "the first individual in the world to be trained by clearly conscious design at the doctoral level for a definite and specific professional objective of working experimentally and clinically with speech and hearing disorders."

Once Travis had completed his doctoral program and received his degree in 1924, Seashore called him a psychologist of psychiatry, just as he had called Bunch a psychologist of otology, and perhaps had called Merry a psychologist of speech, although that title has not been found in any of his writings. Other designations included psychologist of music and psychologist of art.

Seashore's particular talent, George Stoddard[1] wrote in his preface to *Pioneering in Psychology*, was "his ability on crucial occasions to come forward with a plan and a purpose. He combined direct action with an extraordinary power to envisage the shape of things to come." In this

14

particular instance, the crucial occasion was the little girl's problem, the plan was the training of a specialist who might be helpful, and the purpose was to bring that help to the little girl but, more broadly, to bring help to any person who had a problem like hers. What would be involved would be research into the problem and into techniques of therapy, and, in the process, the training of other specialists.

From this time (the early twenties) on, the Program in Speech Pathology was recognized as a distinct entity within the large complex of activities at the University. It was a relatively free-floating unit centered at first in the Departments of Psychology and Speech, gradually moving out of Psychology until it was almost entirely in Speech, then finally becoming a separate department, and in the process constituting a signficant contribution to the establishment and development of the discipline of speech pathology and audiology, as it came to be known.

Travis was ending his first (junior) year at the University when he was chosen by Seashore and Dr. Orton for their special training. He recalls *(15)* that he was pleased to be honored by these gentlemen in this way but that until he was well into his graduate work he was not aware of either the comprehensive plan for the emerging Program or the role he had been assigned in it by his committee.[2] He had been motivated to begin the training primarily because of his enthusiasm for psychology, an enthusiasm he had gained at Graceland College, Lamoni, as a student of Floyd M. McDowell, an Iowa Ph.D. who, in Travis' words, was something of a missionary for psychology.

Travis, who had grown up on a farm in western Nebraska, had gone through the country school's eight grades there and had had one year of high school in the same country school because his Mormon father—a farmer, a teacher, and county superintendent of schools, who had brought up his children on Shakespeare and American history—had taught the teacher, at night, the ninth grade for her to teach his son during the day. After that year Travis had continued his schooling at Lamoni, Iowa, and following the end of his sophomore year at Graceland College had come to The University of Iowa, arriving in Iowa City in June of 1921 with his wife and baby son. He registered as a psychology major. By studying twelve months a year for the next three years he was able to earn his B.A. in 1922, his M.A. in 1923, and his Ph.D. in 1924.

His committee for the doctorate included Seashore, Dr. Orton, Dr. Dean, Edward C. Mabie of Speech, Stephen Bush of Romance Languages, and Gilbert Houser of Biology (Travis had a minor in biology). Mabie served because he was acting head of Speech that year while Merry was on leave to finish his Ph.D. Travis regarded this as "a formidable group. In no way was it a figurehead committee," but one which worked with him closely. Seashore, Dr. Orton, Dr. Dean, and Mabie continued in this relationship even after Travis had his Ph.D.

> I reported to these four people and was guided, even in my research after my degree, by their suggestions. The root of the whole thing began with Seashore. He gave it unity and vitality. Seashore was the leader. He inspired Dr. Orton and Dr. Dean and Mabie. You see, Seashore's very penchant was for creative effort. He was creative and he encouraged us, he supported us. He would do anything for anybody who was doing something original in research.

The Particular Incident. The "particular incident" that Seashore cited as giving "a significant turn of events at the beginning of the cooperation between psychiatry and psychology" seems to have been rather more complicated and more protracted than those words suggest. "Problem" might be a more appropriate term.

The child was Dr. Orton's daughter and her problems apparently were matters of long and deep concern to him. This father, a brilliant and demanding man whose training was in neuropathology, would not accept anything but an organic explanation of her troubles. Everything to him was organic; something physical was wrong, therefore, something was wrong with the brain. That he and Seashore could work together is perhaps an indication of the great stature of both. Certainly their approaches were diametrically opposed, Orton viewing everything as organic, Seashore seeing so many problems as psychological.

The child's problem drew Dr. Orton deeply into a cooperative search with Travis and, in fact, eventually gave Travis his first hypothesis on stuttering to examine. This was the hypothesis that so-called stutterers are different from so-called normal speakers in the dominance pattern of the brain's hemispheres. Studies related to this hypothesis eventually led to the dominance theory, as Travis and Orton named it.

Travis describes Dr. Orton as a good thinker, then adds,

> He had an amazing vocabulary. He could be harsh. But I liked him very much. I emulated him, followed him around for three or four years. I wanted to include him in the dedication of *Speech Pathology* [12]. I dedicated it to Seashore, I wanted to bring Orton in but he said no. He wouldn't allow it. So I mentioned him in the introduction anyway. He was that kind of man. But he ran the hospital very much as a research institution which, of course, suited me fine.

The Individual Plan. The level of scholarship demanded in those days may be inferred from the workings of a loosely defined Plan at Iowa, variously called the Seashore Plan, or the Gifted Student Plan, or the Individual Plan. It was a program devised by Seashore to encourage superior students to range widely in the University, to make scholarly explorations in areas that interested them, and to study in depth and seek some mastery in selected areas that they might choose from the wider field. Each student worked closely with his committee. Examinations were rigorous, and the entire enterprise was demanding in the extreme. The students received small stipends and little cards that admitted them to any class on the campus. They had great privilege and great responsibility.

Travis was in the Plan. So were Wendell Johnson, and others who were to distinguish themselves in the Iowa Program, including Scott Reger and Don Lewis. Reger's professional career has been related intimately to the development of clinical audiometry and the science of audiology, at Iowa and nationally, from 1931, on; Lewis, as a faculty member in the Department of Psychology, made major contributions to the techniques of scaling and was involved in pioneering research with Seashore. Reger *(8)* remembers that early in his days in the Plan he was given a list of sixty books to master. "And master was what was meant. I literally wore the covers off some of them."

Travis, as a student in the Plan, chose to study psychology, biology, psychiatry, neurology, histopathology, physiology, clinical neurology, histology, neuropathology, anatomy twenty hours a week for a year, speech, and even electrical engineering when at one point he needed a special kind of amplifier that nobody seemed to know how to build. With his considerable grounding in both medicine and psychology he later became one of four or five psychologoists in the United States at the time to be members of both the American Physiological Society and the Society for Experimental Biology and Medicine. Also, while still at Iowa, he became a charter member of both the clinical and the counseling divisions of the American Psychological Association.

It has been said *(2)* that at the time the University of Chicago was giving the M.D. degree on the basis of written examinations, Travis could have qualified for that degree with no difficulty. His interest had come to center, perhaps because of his work with Dr. Orton, on electrophysiological procedures and problems, and this in turn had led him to do a great deal of work in the College of Medicine. He recalls that one of his duties, to earn his Individual Plan stipend, was to perform surgery on the brains of dogs so that they could demonstrate a Jacksonian epilepsy for medical students studying under Dr. J. T. McClintock, head of the Department of Physiology in the College of Medicine. He would later do considerable work with animals, especially rats.

Seashore supported the Individual Plan with his vision, his power, and his skill in manipulation. As Travis puts it,

This was Seashore. Seashore set up classes for us in the medical school. We could take anatomy with Dr. Prentiss, neuroanatomy with his understudy who became dean—Dr. MacEwen, we could take physiology with Dr. McClintock, we could take clinical neurology with Dr. Van Epps. We could take psychiatry and neuropathology with Dr. Orton. Seashore did all this. This was an enrichment program that Seashore set up. This was the old man.

Reger *(8)* reports that when

Seashore would call faculty people and ask about psychology students taking a course or about a course being given for them, the heads of the departments often would give the courses themselves. I think again this was an indication of the prestige as well as the power of the Dean. This was tremendous for us because we were getting very fine teaching, you see. And for some reason or other, these gentlemen took pride in doing this sort of thing.

Ruch, and later Lindquist, taught them statistics. Stewart taught acoustics, Seashore himself gave courses for them, and so did the heads of departments in the College of Medicine and the College of Engineering. So did Mabie, and Merry, and other department heads in the College of Liberal Arts. Scholars throughout the entire institution cooperated.

Travis began his research as an undergraduate in the Iowa Psychology Laboratory in the area of voice, a subject in which Seashore had long been interested. Seashore, Travis points out,

had photographed and analyzed voice waves. Ladd and Seashore, of course, had this famous voice laboratory [at Yale] where you could photograph voices with the Dorsey phonelescope. And I picked this up and photographed stutterers' voices under all sorts of conditions. Milton Metfessel was at Iowa then, and Clarence Simon. I was a year ahead of them on my Ph.D. but they were there when I was there and we were always running into each other, borrowing pieces of equipment for whatever we might be building at the time.

Metfessel and Simon received their Ph.D.s in 1925, both in psychology, both under the direction of Seashore. Metfessel's dissertation was on "the technique for objective studies in the vocal art" *(6)*, and Simon's was on "the variability of consecutive wave lengths in vocal and instrumental sounds" *(11)*.

Both men became leaders in their fields, Metfessel in psychology at the University of Southern California, and Simon in speech pathology at Northwestern. Metfessel taught at Iowa for a time after his degree, but Simon returned at once to Northwestern, where he had been a graduate student and where he set about developing a clinical and laboratory center and professional training program in speech rehabilitation. He received Honors of the Association of the American Speech and Hearing Association in 1950.

MAKING THINGS

Travis' comment about borrowing pieces of equipment is not to be taken lightly. Most of the equipment in those days was made on the spot by the student for use in a specific problem. This procedure let the department stretch its equipment money farther than it could have by buying ready-made instruments, and also gave the students considerable training. Seashore, a devoted instrument man, thought that students needed to build their own equipment if they were really to understand what they were doing.

Reger *(8)* recalls well an incident in his first year at Iowa when he was measuring the vibrato of stringed instruments and using an amplifier that had some of the very earliest alternating current radio tubes in it. It was temperamental. It would stop. And when it stopped he had to call Paul Griffith, Travis' assistant, to fix it

> because I knew nothing about it. And sometimes he would be busy and I would have to wait three or four days.
>
> One time when this happened Seashore came down—he came down every week to talk with his students—and wanted to know how things were going and I explained about the amplifier and he said, "Young man, if you expect to be around here very long, don't you think you'd be smart to learn something about your own equipment?" I still remember it. I had already started to take a course in the physics department—Lee Travis took that same course at the same time, the elementary course in electronics. You don't learn how to fix an amplifier as a result of taking one theoretical course. So I talked with Griffith, and asked him what I could do, and he suggested a correspondence course, because he'd had the same experience I did. So even though I'd had about three theoretical courses here, I took a course by correspondence. It was an excellent thing.
>
> They sent equipment, a laboratory manual, and even a soldering iron and some tubes, and an earphone. I had to buy my own batteries. So here I was taking a course by correspondence at the same time I was carrying university work. And I was on Seashore's individual plan. So I was very busy! But I had a wonderful time. It hasn't been work; it's been play. And if I'd inherited a million dollars a few years ago I'd have kept the same job. I might have bought some equipment. There is still some I would like to have.

There are many delightful tales, too, about trying to take laboratory inventory then. Everybody used everything he could get his hands on and it was next to impossible to make out the required University reports of the whereabouts of the bits and pieces the department owned. Seashore often remarked that one of the happiest times in the laboratory came when a given piece of equipment was torn down. That meant it had served its purpose. Another experiment had been finished. It meant too that another student could now pick up the materials thus freed and go one from there.

FLETCHER'S VISIT

For the academic year and summer session preceding Travis' Ph.D. of August 1924, John Fletcher of Tulane was brought to Iowa by Seashore as a visiting professor in psychology. Fletcher was one of the few people in the country then studying stuttering scientifically. As a matter of fact *(3)*, when Seashore and Dr. Orton pooled the techniques and skills of psychology and psychiatry—beginning with the Travis program—the problem of stuttering was being given practically no attention by the academic community at large and such attention as was being given was from more or less self-trained "experts" who, for a fee, promised a "cure."

Travis, who was in Fletcher's seminar, remembers Fletcher as a big, tall man who "stuttered a little bit yet. He was a very fine scholar. He had written a most provocative book, *The Problem of Stuttering (3)*, along purely psychological lines. It was very early and very sound. I'll wager he was the one who inspired me to pick up stuttering as a really important research problem."

In bringing Fletcher to Iowa Seashore obviously was strengthening his scientific program in speech. He may also have been comparing Fletcher with Travis in an effort to choose the man who would continue training as the first "speech pathologist." Travis and others who were there had this impression, Travis from a conversation in which Seashore seemed to be saying this. At any rate, as things worked out Fletcher went back to Tulane and Travis stayed at Iowa.

In his year at Iowa, Fletcher directed the University's first graduate theses concerned exclusively with stuttering, for the 1924 M.A. degrees of Marion McKenzie Font ("A comparison of free-associations of stutterers with those of normal speakers") and Marion Brehm Hebenstreit ("Effect on motor control of negative instruction in the case of stutterers"). Sara Stinchfield Hawk's thesis of 1919 had mentioned stuttering, but it was with these two theses that the Iowa research program in stuttering began in earnest, to continue without interruption to the present.

THE PROGRAM BY 1924

By the fall of 1924, then, the academic requirements had been satisfied for the Bunch, Merry, and Travis doctoral degrees. All three were fundamental to the Iowa Program—Bunch's in what would be audiology, Merry's in speech science, and Travis in the initial research thrust in the area of problems related to speech disorders.

Bunch had continued working with Dr. Dean, conducting hearing tests, instructing residents in the department in the techniques of hearing examinations, and acting as consultant in matters pertaining to the interpretation of hearing tests. By 1924 he and Dr. Dean, singly or jointly, had written eight articles on the significance of pure tone audiometry in otology. The "triumvirate of Seashore, Dean, and Bunch" has been credited *(5)* with giving "the initial impetus to what has developed into audiometric audiology as we know it today."

Merry served as president of the National Association of Teachers of Speech in 1923. In that same year he added Sarah T. Barrows to the faculty of the Speech Department, explaining the importance of this in this note in the November 1923 issue of the *Quarterly Journal of Speech Education* (later *Quarterly Journal of Speech*):

> Among the first American universities to recognize the science of phonetics is the State University of Iowa, which has recently appointed Miss Sarah T. Barrows to a position in phonetics in the Department of Speech. Miss Barrows has studied with many of the foremost phoneticians of Europe, both in theoretical and instrumental phonetics. She is especially interested in comparative phonetics and has studied the sound systems of many different languages. . . . opportunity will be offered for research work in some of the phonetic problems: interpretation of intonation curves, transliteration of dialects, application of phonetics to the teaching of reading. A clinic will be arranged for the improvement of speech difficulties.

The University catalogue for 1923-24 lists the Barrows course under the heading of "speech correction." Miss Barrows *(7)* emphasized auditory stimulation in speech production in contrast to the traditional placement method which had carried over from work with the deaf. She, with Anna D. Cordts, was to publish *The Teacher's Book of Phonetics (1)* in 1926 to support the proposition that "many cases of faulty speech . . . are amenable to remedial measures which the teacher herself may administer." The point is made in an early chapter that modern science has done much for the "comfort and physical well-being of the boys and girls in the public schools . . . But in the case of . . . children who could not learn to read because they could not speak correctly no fore-thought had been taken. No one was trained to meet their needs. The teacher, the nurse, and the parents all lacked knowledge of the technic for correcting their difficulties." The authors go on to observe that "helping the child to normal, distinct speech is a service decidedly worthwhile."

In an introductory statement Miss Barrows and Miss Cordts make "grateful acknowledgement" to several persons, including three who were to figure one way or another in the emerging Program in Speech Pathology, or later in the discipline itself: Ernest Horn and Maude McBroom of the College of Education, and Mildred Freburg (Berry) of the Department of Speech. Freburg moved into speech pathology after she left Iowa. The other two taught courses taken by many in the Program.

Alice Mills, another member of Merry's faculty, taught voice and diction—later voice and phonetics—and is remembered *(10)* by her students as doing a "good bit of work on self-improvement in speech." She emphasized not only artistic considerations but also other factors, for example, voice quality.

One of Seashore's new ideas two or three years earlier had been to section classes according to ability. Merry began to use this idea in the fundamentals course in 1924, with the result that speech problems were given more attention than had been the case before; in fact, little by little, and still rather informally, clinical services were added by the department as part of its basic operating plan. Merry continued, throughout the department, to develop the new scientific approach to speech.

During his doctoral years Travis had published extensively in a wide variety of scientific journals. This, along with Seashore's own very prolific writing, was increasing awareness of the Iowa pioneering in a rather large part of the nation's academic community.

Travis wrote his first article *(13)* before he had his B.A. degree. Among his publications in 1924 were articles based on his research for the M.A. *(14)* and the Ph.D. *(16)*. Years later Travis found himself appalled at the latter, and couldn't remember but felt that Seashore must have approved of the unusual procedure. The fact of the matter was that Travis presented his doctoral dissertation to his committee in the form of reprints. And as far as he knows, or as records indicate, that dissertation is available only in its published version.

THE CLINIC AGAIN

In January of 1924, Seashore's Speech Clinic Committee (Dr. Dean, Dr. Orton, Merry, and Seashore) met with President Jessup to plan for the future. Out of the meeting, according to a memorandum in the Seashore papers in the University archives, came a consensus on five points:

> that we reaffirm the original plan of the organization of the Speech Clinic on the broadest scientific basis through cooperation of the various divisions of the University concerned with the problem;

that we consider the plan of starting a young man who gives promise of achievement in this field through the privilege of a year for research on the ground after he has completed his doctorate;

that Mr. Lee Travis be encouraged to apply for a National Research Council fellowship for the coming academic year with an assignment to work in this field in preparation for the directorship of the Clinic, with the tentative understanding that it is the intention of the University at the present time to appoint him Director of this Clinic with a salary for the first years of about $4,000 for the calendar year, if his work during the research year gives evidence of his fitness for this work, and he feels satisfied to devote himself to this new type of work as a career;

that he be encouraged to begin at once to organize his work through studies in phonetics and practical contact with actual cases, and that a trainer for routine work to cooperate with him be secured as soon as possible; and

that temporarily he may operate from the Psychological Clinic, but that it be our aim to secure special quarters for the Speech Clinic as soon as possible.

This word was passed on to Travis a few months before he received his Ph.D. degree, and he proceeded to apply for an NRC postdoctoral fellowship. Seashore and E. L. Thorndike of Columbia were leaders in affairs of the Council at that time. The fellowship was granted and Travis was given an office and laboratory space in the outpatient area of the Psychopathic Hospital.

Apparently to enhance the idea of cooperation between Psychology and Psychiatry, Seashore let it be assumed from Travis' presence in the hospital that the Travis program was part of the Department of Psychiatry. Of course it was, in a measure. But it was primarily in the Department of Psychology. And it was the core of what there was by then of the Iowa Program in Speech Pathology.

REFERENCES

1. Sarah T. Barrows and Anna D. Cordts, *The Teacher's Book of Phonetics* (New York: Ginn and Company, 1933).

2. Bryng Bryngelson, taped conversation with author, Minneapolis, February 27, 1968.

3. John Fletcher, *The Problem of Stuttering* (New York: Longmans, Green, 1928).

4. Wendell Johnson (Ed.), *Stuttering in Children and Adults* (Minneapolis: University of Minnesota Press, 1955).

5. Dean Lierle (with Scott Reger), "The Origin and Development of

Audiometric Audiology at the University of Iowa," *Transactions of the American Otological Society, 54,* 1966, 19-23.

6. Milton F. Metfessel, "The Technique for Objective Studies of the Vocal Art," *Psychological Monographs, 36,* 1927, 1-40.

7. Bessie Rasmus (Petersen), conversation with author, Iowa City, April 10, 1968.

8. Scott Reger, taped conversation with author, Iowa City, April 3, 1968.

9. Carl E. Seashore, *Pioneering in Psychology* (Iowa City: University of Iowa Press, 1942).

10. Dorothy Sherman, conversation with author, Iowa City, April 1968.

11. Clarence T. Simon, "The Variability of Consecutive Wavelengths in Vocal and Instrumental Sounds," *Psychological Monographs, 36,* 1927, 41-83.

12. Lee Edward Travis, *Speech Pathology* (New York: D. Appleton-Century, 1931).

13. Lee Edward Travis, "Studies in Dissociation, Changes in the Auditory Threshold Induced by 'Crystal Gazing,' " *Journal of Experimental Psychology, 5,* October 1922, 338-346.

14. Lee Edward Travis, "Suggestibility and Negativism as Measured by Auditory Threshold during Reverie," *Journal of Abnormal Psychology, 18,* January 1924, 350-368.

15. Lee Edward Travis, taped conversation with author, Los Angeles, February 8, 1968.

16. Lee Edward Travis, "Test for Distinguishing between Schizophrenoses and Psychoneuroses," *Journal of Abnormal and Social Psychology, 19,* October-December 1924, 283-298.

NOTES

[1] Stoddard, with an Iowa Ph.D. (1925) in psychology, served on the University faculty from 1928 to 1942. In chronological order, his positions were Acting Director of the Child Welfare Research Station, Director of the Station, Dean of the Graduate College, and head of the Department of Psychology, the latter post being held concurrently with the deanship in the 1938-39 academic year.

[2] Where the source is clear, interview material and material from personal correspondence are keyed to the reference list only once within each chapter, on initial use.

3

THE TRAVIS PERIOD: NRC—1924-1927

Lee Travis' NRC fellowship was twice renewed, with the result that for the three years, 1924-1927, he had Council support of $200 a month and a full-time commitment to research. In addition, he taught courses in both the Speech and Psychology departments and directed graduate work even though he held no official position for doing either. In the sense that history is the biography of leaders, the fellowship time was a prelude to the beginning of the Travis period. That period was to continue some 14 years from 1924, when the fellowship was first granted.

For the academic year 1924-25 Travis was listed in the University catalogue as a member of the Psychology faculty, teaching a two-hour course in the clinical psychology of speech. The catalogue description called the course "a critical and practical survey of the theories of *speech pathology* [italics ours] with clinical practice designed as a fundamental course for those who are to practice or teach corrective speech." This may be the first appearance in print of the term "speech pathology," and the first course ever offered in "speech pathology."

The term "speech pathology" first began to appear during the twenties, and has been attributed by some to Seashore. Travis *(12)* has the feeling that it wasn't coined deliberately by anybody. It is Travis' suggestion that in his own student work in the College of Medicine, where he was studying various pathologies, he might well have drifted into using the phrase quite naturally, referring to yet another pathology. He says he can't recall hearing anyone else use it before he began to, so he may have been the first. Obviously he didn't consider it an important point, for when he called his 1931 book *Speech Pathology (11)* he made no mention of anything special about the term.

Psychology offerings for 1924-1925 included a course related to the emerging Program, a seminar in the "psychology of music and speech" taught by Milton Metfessel. The course was "designed primarily for advanced students interested in scientific aspects of music and speech from a psychological viewpoint." And in the summer of 1924, the Speech Department's "speech correction" grouping was "offered conjointly by the Department of Speech and the Child Welfare Research Station, with the cooperation of other departments and colleges of the University." Sarah Barrows is given as the instructor, and the catalogue description of one of her courses is "a study of difficulty which children have in English speech, exclusive of stuttering and neurotic speech disorders; how to make a speech diagnosis, drills for correction. Students will be given the opportunity to observe and assist in the Speech Clinic."

In 1925-1926 seven courses were listed in the Speech Department's sequence in voice science. It was not until the year 1926-27 that another speech pathology course appeared. It was called speech correction, was offered in the Speech Department, and was taught by Travis and Bessie Rasmus; it included "clinical practice" and was described as "a fundamental course in speech correction for majors in the department who intend to teach." The Metfessel seminar in the psychology of music and speech continued during these years.

HISTORIC MEETINGS OF 1925

The year 1925 was an historic one in this NRC fellowship period because it was then that two meetings of major importance to both the Iowa Program and the discipline of speech pathology were held on the Iowa campus. Dean Carl E. Seashore felt that Travis was well enough known that the University might appropriately host a conference of a selected group of professional people who were conversant with methods of science and were interested in the problem of speech disorders. Travis *(12)* liked the idea, and proceeded to

> round up eight or ten people and Seashore paid their way here. And we had a conference and they slept on cots in the outpatient department at the Psychopathic Hospital and in our homes. We had Muyskens of Michigan, Robert West of Wisconsin, Smiley Blanton of Minnesota [see *Asha, 9,* January 1967, 9], Pauline Camp of the Wisconsin public schools, Meyer Solomon, a psychiatrist from Chicago, Sara Stinchfield Hawk, G. Oscar Russell of Ohio State, maybe two or three others. We had phoneticians, psychiatrists, psychologists, speech people, two or three M.D.s. And we talked for a couple of days, mainly about speech disorders and research. And at the end of the conference we went out to my house [513 South Summit Street] and decided we'd organize.

West, who had been at Iowa before going to Wisconsin, took the organizing idea to the convention of the National Association of Teachers of Speech that fall—"we all belonged to that Association" Travis explains—and actually organized the new group there and became its first president. It was called the American Academy of Speech Correction[1] and, after going through two name changes, in 1947 became the American Speech and Hearing Association. Hayes Newby *(8)* recounted much of this in his 1964 presidential address at the ASHA convention. Travis tried unsuccessfully to get the word "study" in the original name because, as he puts it, "I thought we should have it modest. We were just starting." (In 1927, the title *was* changed to the "American Society for the Study of Disorders of Speech" and remained so for seven years.)

Bryng Bryngelson, who had been at Iowa earlier and had returned in 1922 to head the speech fundamentals program and to do graduate work with Travis, recalls *(1)* that he and Mrs. Bryngelson (Arminda Mowre) were guests at the Travis home for the historic meeting. And when graduate students were admitted to the Association, Bryngelson was among the first.

The second of the two historic conferences of 1925 was sponsored by the University of Iowa Extension Division, with E. C. Mabie of the Speech Department in charge. The importance of this conference, as Bryngelson sees it, was that it marked the beginning of a development which in the thirties would bring the separation, at the national level, of speech pathology from general speech.

One particularly dramatic session revealed something of the attitude held in those days by certain educators toward research involving human subjects. Mabie arranged to have a number of out-of-town speech people here and devoted one of the three major conference sessions to a consideration of research. Alice Mills presided. Iowa's Milton Metfessel and Giles W. Gray demonstrated and discussed a technique for the experimental study of voice and speech. West of Wisconsin, an associate in public speaking in the Iowa Speech Department in 1920-21, reported on an investigation in the nature of vocal sound. Sarah Barrows spoke on the application of phonetics to problems of speech correction. Finally, Travis reported on a study he had done on "muscular fixation of the stutterer's voice under emotion." This had been published two months earlier in *Science (62*, August 28, 1925, 207-8).

In this study he had photographed, by use of the phonelescope, voices of stutterers and nonstutterers singing "ah" under four conditions: in a unemotional situation, after being closely questioned, after going into a darkened room and having a pistol fired near them, and after receiving an electric shock. He had expected to find greater variability under emotion in the pitch of the stutterers than in that of the nonstutterers but actually found the opposite. He concluded that "instead of the emotional upheaval producing a muscular lability in the case of the stutterer, it produced a muscular fixation wherein the muscular balance that was taken to produce the 'ah' was rigidly maintained."

After Travis had finished, Bryngelson remembers, James M. O'Neill of Wisconsin "stood up and gave the worst tirade on research that I have ever heard. 'To think,' he said, 'of making a rat out of a human being and surprising him in a dark room by shooting a pistol in his ear!' " And apparently others felt the same way because O'Neill's comments were seconded with spirit. The new psychology apparently was still too new for some.

Bryngelson also remembers another incident at the end of the same day through which, as a matter of fact, the course of events led to his first position, with O'Neill and West at Wisconsin. It was after a dinner that evening when discussion turned to mental testing. Bryngelson tells it this way:

> I was only a graduate student and I was shaking like a leaf and I don't know how I got the nerve but I stood up and said, "I doubt very much that you can get an adequate IQ on an individual who is emotionally disturbed," and I sat down. Seashore told me afterward that was the best statement of the evening.
>
> O'Neill asked Seashore who I was. Later O'Neill offered me this position and I accepted. Then I asked him how he had chosen me and he answered he had liked my statement but more than that he had never heard such a euphonious name as Bryng Bryngelson! Nobody could have a name like that!

THE UNIVERSITY BULLETIN

Relations of the Department of Psychology to other departments and services at the University were graphically presented to the people of the state of Iowa in the June 25, 1926 issue of the University's Bulletin in this drawing which was used for the cover design:

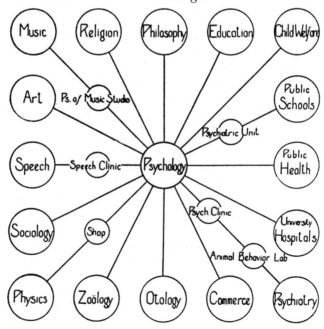

The entire issue was given over to a detailing of the work within the Department of Psychology and in its interdisciplinary enterprises with other departments and services. The text supported the message of the cover drawing, namely, that Psychology was very much in the center of things and related to a large sector of the University.

THE GROWTH OF SPEECH SCIENCE

In the years of the Travis NRC fellowship, as for almost a decade before, the emphasis on research in the Department of Psychology was matched in the Department of Speech in the innovative program in speech science established and nurtured by Glenn Merry, who by then had considerably strengthened the total program in the Department of Speech. Feeling that the time had come when his department could offer the Ph.D. degree, he discussed the matter with Seashore, only to discover that there was a distressing difference of opinion. Merry expected that the degree would be granted by the Speech Department. Seashore said that that department was not strong enough and that the degree should be granted by, and also directed by, a stronger department, which in many cases would be the Department of Psychology. The latter view prevailed and Merry resigned. He left Iowa for Harvard in 1926.

Mabie, whom Merry had brought in to teach theater, succeeded him as head of the department, and proceeded to give strong support to Merry's speech science program even though his own training and interest were in theater. Like Merry, he supported research at the national level too. As president of the National Association of the Teachers of Speech, following Merry, he initiated the plan for special research issues of the *Quarterly Journal of Speech Education* (see the April 1926 issue, pp. 203-4) and it was by his action that a national committee on research was named. Travis was a member, as were Windsor P. Daggett of New York and A. M. Drummond of Cornell University. One of Mabie's first appointments after he became department head was that of Charles Woolbert, a pioneer in the behavioristic approach to speech, who came to Iowa from Illinois to succeed Bryngelson as head of the speech fundamentals program. Woolbert's work at Iowa has been described as brief and brilliant. There are those who feel *(4)* that the program he envisaged would have made an important contribution to the field, but it was not carried on by others when he died and has not been developed since.

Woolbert in turn brought a former colleague, Giles Gray, from Illinois to Iowa. Gray, a few years later, would publish *Bases of Speech (3)*, one of the new scientifically oriented texts to be written in this period. (Gray's Ph.D. was granted in 1926. Seashore directed his research, which was on the vibrato in speech; Travis and Metfessel were on his committee. His thesis was published in book form *[2]* by the National Association of the Teachers of Speech.)

Seashore (*10,* p. 12) had warm words for Mabie:

> Mabie had had no advanced training in laboratory psychology but saw very clearly the possibilities involved in my plan and entered enthusiastically upon a program of developing the department along these lines, largely in cooperation with psychology, his own field being dramatic art. This broadening of the base for the department immediately gave it great strength and attracted students of high quality into graduate work. Naturally, since methods of acoustics and their application, and to some extent phonetics, had been developed in the psychological laboratory, it was agreed that the department of speech should have full privileges in sharing this laboratory for research, and candidates for the doctorate who approached speech from the scientific side would be largely under the direction of a psychologist. Here came in such men as Metfessel, [Joseph] Tiffin, [Don] Lewis, [Grant] Fairbanks and [Milton] Cowan for pioneering leadership in the conduct of research. In planning research projects, special attention was given to the effort to evaluate all forms of transfer of developments in the psychology of music in so far as they could be applied to the psychology of speech and linguistics.
>
> With the work of Metfessel came our development of photographic procedures to take the place of the graphic method followed by Merry. This immediately led to great expansion and variety of techniques, opening up new possibilities for ready and accurate measurement in speech and music. Here came the phono-photostrobograph and a variety of oscillographic techniques leading to the studies of harmonic analysis.

The work Seashore mentions was being carried on, as he states, in the Psychological Laboratory. But toward the end of the twenties a Speech Department Laboratory was added. Metfessel did much of the work of developing that Laboratory as well as a laboratory course which was required of all speech majors.

THE LABORATORY

The main emphasis for Travis in this period was on another laboratory, the one which he designed, and with his associates quite literally had built, in the basement of the Psychopathic Hospital. As Johnson (*6,* p. 7) later explained, it was out of this laboratory that the Speech Clinic and the University's present research, clinical, and professional training program in speech pathology and audiology developed;

> The fact that the program began substantially with the building of a laboratory was aptly symbolic of the fundamental Seashorian thinking

that has so deeply affected the work in speech pathology and audiology at Iowa from the beginning. Dean Seashore's point of view—effectively fostered also, and crucially after Dean Seashore's retirement, by Professor Mabie—was that before a service can be rendered men and women must be properly trained to render it, before they can be properly trained there must be dependable knowledge and methods to be imparted to them, and before there can be dependable knowledge and methods there must be scientific research. In other words, there must be productive laboratories before there can be worthwhile classrooms, and there must be worthwhile classrooms before there can be effective clinics.

So it was that in Dean Seashore's particular way of putting first things first, the Iowa Program in Speech Pathology and Audiology was begun, not by building a clinic or a school, but by training a research worker and designing a laboratory.

Travis and Dr. Orton. During Travis' postdoctoral years he and Dr. Orton were much involved in their search for an understanding of speech problems, especially those of Dr. Orton's daughter. Travis recalls that as Dr. Orton studied her clinically he

> ran across her reversals. So he pursued this and got a grant for the Psychopathic Hospital from the Rockefeller people, a two-year grant, to study reading disability. And he hired research staff members. Among them interestingly was a neuroanatomist. She would make sections of the right and left side of the nervous system all the way from the cord to the cortex, checking for an unequal distribution in space and in numbers of nerve cells to see if there was an anatomical basis for cerebral dominance. He had Loretta Bender as a medical student. She went into the reading end. He wanted to look at speech too and because I was a National Research Council fellow then in the hospital he asked me if I would take the research in speech and that's how that started.

The Mobile Clinic. The Orton grant made possible a mobile mental hygiene clinic which traveled over the state and which, in combination with the program on campus, constituted a major enterprise. At least four historical documents in the archives of the Psychopathic Hospital describe phases of the work. The entire February 13, 1926 issue (*10:* 7) of the *University of Iowa Service Bulletin* was given over to this project. The March 1926 issue (*4:* 3) of the *Mental Hygiene Bulletin* carried an article entitled "Mobile Mental Hygiene Clinic in Iowa." The October 1926 (*10:* 4) issue of *Mental Hygiene* included an article by June F. Lyday on "The Green County Mental Clinic." The fourth document (no author listed) is the report of the "Research Program of the Mobile and Laboratory Units of the Iowa State Psychopathic Hospital Carried out Under a Grant from the Rockefeller Foundation January 1926-October 1927."

Personnel of the laboratory unit, as listed in that report (p. 23) are:

Dr. Samuel T. Orton, director; Miss June F. Lyday, research associate and executive assistant; Dr. Ada Potter, research professor in neuroanatomy and neuropathology; Mr. Lee E. Travis, national research council fellow in biological sciences; Miss Marion Monroe, research associate in psychology; Dr. Loretta Bender, research associate in cerebral physiology; Miss Bessie Rasmus, research assistant in speech correction; Miss Della Pepler, technician; Miss Charlotte Fisk, secretary, succeeded by Mrs. Peggy Torrance.

Miss Lyday and Dr. Orton were married some time after they left Iowa City. Miss Fisk became a pediatrician and went into practice in Des Moines. Miss Rasmus became Mrs. William J. Petersen of Iowa City. She *(9)* recalls that Don Durrell, who later headed a reading clinic in Boston, gave the psychological tests in the Orton enterprise. Secretaries, in addition to Miss Fisk, included Dorothy McGlone, who became Mrs. Willard Lampe of Iowa City, and Mrs. Yorke Herren, whose husband was one of Travis' early students.

In one section of the report (pp. 26, 27), "Studies in Speech Disorders" are described as follows:

In September 1925, Mr. Travis began work under the direction of Dr. Orton upon the problem of stuttering, as a Fellow of the National Research Council. The approach to this field has been largely physiological, and kymographic studies of dysintegration of the breathing musculature during stuttering, phonophotographic studies of the stutterer's voice and studies of the reflexes during stuttering were undertaken in the fall of 1925. After the organization of the Laboratory Unit, Mr. Travis' work was coordinated with the program centering about the problem of cerebral dominance and this attack applied to stuttering has already yielded results of great promise.

The laboratory work has included the perfection of apparatus with radio amplification for the registration of action currents and motor studies of handedness. Retraining experiments based on these findings have been tried at the Hospital with a small group of stutterers and have resulted in great improvement in individual cases. In September 1927, Mr. Travis was appointed Psychologist to the Psychopathic Hospital and Director of the Speech Clinic and he will continue his experimental work during the year. Reports upon his findings will appear in the *Archives of Neurology and Psychology* and elsewhere. . . .

Miss Rasmus assisted at the Hospital and in the field by giving special examinations in over 200 cases with articulatory speech defects, by outlining in detail methods for their correction, by demonstrating these methods to the teachers, and by undertaking retraining herself in a number of cases. She also served as assistant to Miss Monroe in the examination and training of the reading cases.

Cerebral Dominance. Travis remembers that very early in the grant program Dr. Orton

> got the idea that what is wrong with stutterers is a lack of sufficient cerebral dominance. Now he didn't know too much about theory, if there was a theory, and this was the first I'd heard of it. So I commenced to research it in mirror writing, in studies of handedness of people. I had done my first work on stuttering and the voice at Schaeffer Hall so now I went on with it at the Psychopathic Hospital or Clinic with the kymograph where I got breathing records, movements of the larynx, and that type of thing. Orton had this equipment built for me, a beautiful kymograph. Freund, a German technician, built it right there in the hospital. Oh, it was worth a thousand dollars then.
>
> It was because of my new interest in handedness that I went on to develop action current equipment so I could find out which side got the nerve impulses first in squeezing the hands or in movement or whatever I was studying. I wanted to get behind gross movement. Physiologists were recording gross muscle contraction but I thought if I could get evidences of muscular contraction through such things as electrical currents, how much better.

Electrical Potential. And Travis interests ranged farther.

> I had read about this, about the electrical potential from muscles so I went to [A. N.] Ford, the head of Electrical Engineering at Iowa, at the time, and I asked him to help me develop apparatus for picking up these electrical currents from the contraction of muscles. And he did. He got intrigued by it. And he gave me a young man by the name of Ted Hunter. [This would be 1926.]
>
> Seashore hired Ted Hunter for me. Dean Seashore would give me almost anything he could. So he gave me Ted Hunter [later with the Hunter Manufacturing Company of Coralville, makers of electronic equipment, and for many years before that an instrument man for the Psychology Department] and we developed this muscle action potential equipment. And all I wanted to do was study cerebral dominance. I wanted to measure the appearance in muscle of nerve impulses from the two sides, arms, legs, the masseter muscles of the jaws.

BUILDING THE LABORATORY

We had two other rooms down there in the basement, the wing toward the Children's Hospital. One of these rooms had a door but no window. Absolutely no light, no air, no nothing, in it. And we used to work in there until we would almost faint. Ted and I would work in there 12 and 14 and 16 hours a day, in that room, not a bit of air, just a little door that went out into the hall, all artificial lights. Why, I can remember having the blind staggers, because we'd been so absorbed, you see, building this equipment. And we'd discover things as we went along, for example, take this voice wave. You see, Seashore was recording voices on this Dorsey phonelescope. Well I got the idea of using the Dorsey phonelescope for the action potentials, for tremors, and everything. Here was a piece of equipment that I could adapt and I had electrical currents going through this thing the same as we had voice waves going through it.

In the equipment we were building I wanted to record the action potentials from the two arms but I didn't want any cross talk. Well, this was quite a trick electrically in those days. So Ted and I did that by broadcasting. We broadcast at different carrier lengths and ran those from the right arm on one and those from the left arm on another carrier wave. We had the most complicated arrangement you ever saw. That room was absolutely full of condensers, transformers, tubes, wires, batteries. And we had to have all this equipment in order to be sure that one arm wasn't picking up the other one through the body. We really broadcast those action potentials and then picked them up through receivers. As far as I know we were the first people in America to record action potentials from muscles.

Hunter *(5)* remembers those times as the most exciting in his long experience in research; as a matter of fact, they may have made an important difference in the direction of his life work. He went on from the University to spend many years in the field, distinguishing himself as an electrical engineer, but then decided that too much of his effort was being spent on projects related to war and killing, and that he would prefer to involve himself again, as in the Travis period, in the more creative enterprise of developing instruments for measurements in the study of human problems. And so, although by then he was a prominent engineer in his own right, with a position of high responsibility in industry, and with membership on the board of directors of the prestigious Institute of Electrical and Electronic Engineers, he chose in 1945 to return to the University to head the instrument shop for the Department of Psychology. And there he continued to work until his retirement in 1963, remaining active even after that, but from then on in the affairs of the Hunter Manufacturing Company of Coralville, makers of electronic equipment.

When he thinks back to the time he was working with Travis he recalls how jammed full of equipment that basement room became. "When you're in a new area," he explains, when you're doing research work, you generally wind up to be a messer. You won't give up anything that has worked for you previously. You want to try the new thing but you want to keep the old in case you have to go back. So, as a result, you collect a lot of things.

The big problem we had at that time was in the fact that we were trying to operate with amplifying action potentials in a room where you had a very considerable amount of electrical disturbance from the electrical circuits. We would have to wait until most of the circuits were not being used so as to avoid the disturbance.

So they often worked late at night while the rest of the hospital was asleep. Hunter remembers that when they rigged up the apparatus to broadcast the waves they picked them up with a radio receiver and amplified them and recorded them.

We put the tubes inside of a box and hung them from the ceiling on screen door springs and had them almost completely isolated from the noise of the room. We recorded them on an oscilloscope, one of the early instruments in the game. This was how we were able to get these things recorded at that time. It was pioneering then. We developed a camera. I actually made that thing. And we had a special method for developing the film. We took pictures of different kinds of action potential waves of those who were stutterers and those who were not.

Hunter recalls that they worked with many people in the hospital complex. Once, for example, for Iowa's renowned orthopedic surgeon, Dr. Arthur Steindler, they recorded action potentials in a particular nerve fiber leading to the ear of a cat because that was a point of interest in research Dr. Steindler was doing at the time.

And there was a series of studies Hunter remembers with some glee. It had to do with action potentials in the presence and absence of alcohol.

We didn't have much of a problem in getting alcohol at the time, even though those were prohibition days, because we had the hospital to draw from, and we had no trouble at all getting students who were willing to be subjects. And the results were just as you might expect. With alcohol, the nerve wave looked very much like that of a frog. So I guess the moral is, drink a lot of alcohol if you want to go back all the way.

Some of the Travis students had duties as nursemaids or chaperons, or whatever the word would be, for the subjects. And there were delicate matters of concern such as whether a nurse should be in attendance when the experimenters attached electrodes to the legs of female subjects. These were serious problems at the time even if they are now remembered with a smile.

As the experimentation proceeded, Hunter and Travis managed to refine some of their equipment to a certain extent and then it wasn't too long, a matter of four or five years, as Hunter points out,

> before they began to develop vacuum tubes that would do the job quite well. Now, of course, we have transistors and they are not bothered by vibrations and so this problem should be rather easy.
>
> We were primarily in the business of recording action potentials and I remember very distinctly one thing that happened. By using the then modern techniques of amplifying the waves, we put these out over radio station WSUI as a broadcast of nerve potentials. And this received great acclaim clear across the nation in the news. The New York Times carried it. For the first time nerve currents were broadcast over a radio station.

PUBLIC RELATIONS

This broadcast suggests that Travis may have taken his cue on public relations and publications from Seashore, who more often than not in his voluminous writing appeared outside the field of psychology. Metfessel, in a biography of Seashore in 1950 *(7)*, mentions that only a small part of Seashore's very considerable writing was done for standard psychological journals.

> When he wrote on a subject of interest to several sciences, he published his work in *Science* and *The Scientific Monthly*. Other contributions were made directly in the channels of the field to which psychological methods were applied. . . . His style was lucid and affirmative, and in his nontechnical writing he used the first person with conversational freedom. . . . He cooperated with the public press, and welcomed interviews with newspapermen on programs, projects, and specific studies.

A sampling of the Program's public relations work was saved in a scrapbook kept by Mrs. Betty Walker, secretary to Travis and the Psychological and Speech Clinic in the thirties. She clipped a number of articles from the popular press and kept these in the book which in 1968 she presented to the Department of Speech Pathology and Audiology for its archive collection. In her clippings are the usual items about meetings and appointments and programs. There are also others that are definitely not routine. There is one, for example, on artist Grant Wood's brain waves. There is another on a study of handedness in rats. One is about stutterers playing left-handed ping-pong to help their speech. And there's a "wanted" one, too: Wanted—100 Stutterers. The item, dated December 1934, explained that the Speech Department was starting a research project and wanted to find "at least 100 stutterers who will submit to free treatment and examination by speech experts."

Travis and the Program were becoming widely known. He *(12)* explains,

Some of the things I did I published in *Science*. These hit the press. Several things hit the press, mostly about stuttering. And then I got to be in demand talking. And I would talk about the research we were doing. And so people began to come from all over, not only from Iowa but from the whole country. Generally, I would say we would have 25 stutterers all the time around there that we could use in research. And then when we needed more I would drive out around Iowa City, to the homes of people who had sent word to me or of whom I'd heard, and ask them to come in to serve as subjects. Almost from the beginning our research involved statistical procedures but we didn't have nearly as good statistical methods for the treatment of small samples as we have now so we had to get a lot of people. So I guess you could say I was always hunting for stutterers.

BRAIN WAVES

To complete his training under the National Research Council fellowship, Travis spent the final six months of his three years visiting laboratories and clinics in Berlin, Hamburg, London, and Utrecht. In Utrecht he studied with the renowned Dutch physiologist, Hendrik Zwaardemaker, to learn more about certain electrophysiological procedures than he had been able to on his own in his laboratory in the Psychopathic Hospital. He wanted to know how to record brain waves as well as action potential currents. This was his new interest.

REFERENCES

1. Bryng Bryngelson, taped conversation with author, Minneapolis, February 27, 1968.

2. Giles Wilkeson Gray, *An Experimental Study of the Vibrato in Speech* (Madison: National Association of Teachers of Speech, 1926), hardcover offprint from *Quarterly Journal of Speech Education, 12,* November 1926, 296-333.

3. Giles Wilkeson Gray and Claude Merton Wise, *Bases of Speech* (New York: Harper, 1934, revised edition 1946).

4. Ernest Henrikson, taped conversation with author, Minneapolis, February 27, 1968.

5. Theodore Hunter, taped conversation with author, Coralville, April 4, 1968, and correspondence, March 2, 1972.

6. Wendell Johnson (Ed.), *Stuttering in Children and Adults* (Minneapolis: University of Minnesota Press, 1955).

7. Milton Metfessel, "Carl Emil Seashore, 1866-1949," *Science, 3,* 1950, 713-717.

8. Hayes Newby, "Reflections on Becoming Forty," *Asha, 7,* January 1965, 3-7.

9. Bessie Rasmus Petersen, conversation with author, Iowa City, April 10, 1968.

10. Carl Emil Seashore, *Pioneering in Psychology* (Iowa City: University of Iowa Press, 1942).

11. Lee Edward Travis, *Speech Pathology* (New York: D. Appleton-Century, 1931).

12. Lee Edward Travis, taped conversation with author, Los Angeles, February 8, 1968.

NOTE

[1] Charter members of the American Academy of Speech Correction, the organization which now is the American Speech and Hearing Association, as listed in the records of that association were: Margaret Blanton, Smiley Blanton, Richard Bordon, Frederick Brown, Alvin Busse, Pauline Camp, Eudora Estabrook, Sina Fladeland, Mabel Gifford, Max Goldstein, Ruth Green, Elmer Kenyon, Mabel Lacy, Thyrza Nickols, Samuel Robbins, Sara Stinchfield, Jane Taylor, C. K. Thomas, Lee Edward Travis, Lavilla Ward, Robert West, and Jane Dorsey Zimmerman.

4

THE TRAVIS PERIOD: People and Climate

In the Travis period, The University of Iowa became "a mecca for graduate students" who were interested in the pioneering being done here in the scientific study of speech and speech disabilities. They made up a "remarkable group." Thus Seashore (*11*, p. 135) wrote, describing the scene: "while Lee Travis was still a student, people began coming to Iowa to work with him; they continued coming, and in increasing numbers, after he had received the Ph.D., on through the three fellowship years, then throughout the time when he was officially the administrator of the Iowa Program in Speech Pathology."

Seashore, who was writing in 1942, paired his estimate of the situation and the students with a survey made in the late thirties. At that time, according to his survey, Iowa-trained people were heading four of the country's five well-established speech clinics of university rank, and two-thirds of the rest of the nation's scientifically oriented clinics. These latter were not as highly developed as the other five, but were using the so-called Iowa pattern of scientific investigation of the nature of speech and speech problems.

Margaret Hall Powers (*9*) recalls that when she came to Iowa to study with Travis she found "an environment of lively inquiry which Seashore may have created but which Travis certainly maintained and greatly augmented." In her opinion, "it is not accidental that Travis people fanned out and became leaders everywhere. Of course this began to change as Iowa people's graduates went on into colleges and universities; the Iowa influence was somewhat diluted as it became second and third generation. But there was a period when practically all the work was coming out of Iowa and the people were coming out of Iowa."

Had Seashore been writing in 1968 (the final year of the period of this book) he might have suggested that the roster of recipients of the Honors of the Association award of the American Speech and Hearing Association, and likewise the roster of Association presidents, provided other indications of the Iowa leadership. In 1968 there were thirty-two names on the Honors roster. Twelve of those are Iowa alumni or faculty.[1] Eight of the twelve are Travis students: Wendell Johnson, Delyte Morris, Grant Fairbanks, Margaret Hall Powers, Charles Van Riper, Mack D. Steer, Bryng Bryngelson, and Herbert Koepp-Baker, honored in that order. The other four from Iowa are Seashore and three of his students. Seashore won the award in 1944, the first year it was given; Travis won it in 1947; Clarence T. Simon, in 1950; and Sara Stinchfield Hawk, in 1953. Hawk worked closely also with Bird T. Baldwin, director of the Child Welfare Research Station. She had completed her study at Iowa before Travis came; Simon had followed him by a year for the Ph.D.

The roster of presidents of the Association, as of 1968, also carried thirty-two names. Again, twelve of the individuals so named have the Ph.D. from Iowa. And six of the twelve are Travis students: Bryngelson, Koepp-Baker, Morris, Johnson, Steer, and Powers, in office in that order. The other six are Travis, whose term was 1935-36; Hawk, 1939-40; Simon, 1946; James F. Curtis, 1962; Hayes A. Newby, 1964; and Duane C. Spriestersbach, 1965. As a matter of fact, Curtis was on campus and in the Program in the Travis era but is not included here as a Travis student since at that time, as a high school teacher, he was in Iowa City only for Saturday classes, was not a degree candidate, and studied not with Travis but with Johnson and with Harry Barnes, head of the speech fundamentals course. So discussion of Curtis' work appears to be more appropriate in later periods, when he began a degree program and went on to become the first head of the Iowa Department of Speech Pathology and Audiology.

In terms of the future of the new discipline, there was such richness in the personnel in the Iowa Program in early years that the class rolls were later described as a Who's Who. Though that statement may well be an exaggeration, a pause is indicated in this recounting of events simply to see who was among those present and what the climate was like. Several of the individuals introduced here will, of course, appear again as the story unfolds.

One way to begin introductions is with the Travis students on the ASHA Honors list. In the chronology of initial contact with the Iowa Program, Bryngelson came first, then Johnson, then Van Riper, Steer, Fairbanks, Morris, Powers, and Koepp-Baker.

Bryngelson had been a fellow in the Iowa Speech Department in 1921, and had later returned to head the speech fundamentals program and to work with Travis for the M.S. degree, which he received in 1926. His thesis for this was the third study at Iowa to deal exclusively with stuttering. He then taught at Wisconsin and Minnesota, came back to Iowa in 1930, finished his Ph.D. in 1931, and returned to the University of Minnesota where he developed clinical programs within the University's speech and hospital areas, and at the Veterans Administration hospital. He was administrative head of these for many years, becoming emeritus in the sixties. He is the author of a number of books and many articles. In addition to his service as ASHA president, he was the Association's treasurer from 1933 to 1942.

Johnson came to Iowa in 1926 as a junior in English. He stuttered so severely that at times he was all but speechless, though he had managed to finish two years of work at McPherson College, McPherson, Kansas. There he had found an understanding English teacher, Florence E. Teager, who not only brought him to the point of speaking in class but also—when she felt he was ready—told him of Travis' research and encouraged him to come to Iowa. (She had been a student here, came back for her Ph.D. in 1931, taught at the University of Illinois, and made her home in Cedar Rapids after retirement.)

Miss Teager recalls *(13)* that Johnson "seemed to come alive at the idea" that he try Iowa. She remembers him as eager and determined. When he stopped to visit her in Des Moines on his way to Iowa City "he was happy, relaxed." He was fond of explaining *(6)* later that he came to Iowa to get his stuttering "cured" and became a speech pathologist because he needed one. He received his B.A. in 1928, his M.A. in 1929, and his Ph.D. in 1931. He later assumed administrative responsibilities in the University Speech Clinic, became chairman of the University's Council on Speech Pathology and Audiology, and through prolific writing and extensive lecturing became known as a world authority on stuttering and as a leading figure in general semantics. He was the next person after Seashore to win the Honors of the Association award of ASHA. He spent his entire professional career as a member of the University of Iowa faculty, first with a triple appointment in Psychology, Speech, and Child Welfare, then with a joint appointment in Speech Pathology and Psychology. He became a research assistant in 1930, a member of the faculty in 1937. In 1963 he was named Louis W. Hill Research Professor. He died in 1965.

Van Riper was brought to Iowa by Bryngelson in 1930, when Bryngelson returned to complete his Ph.D. Van Riper, just after completing his M.A. in English at the University of Michigan, had gone to Minneapolis to ask Bryngelson to help him with his stuttering problem. Bryngelson told him he was soon to leave for Iowa City, invited him to accompany him, Van Riper accepted, and so for the next year the two men lived and worked together in Iowa City. Van Riper became so interested in what was going on at Iowa that he undertook graduate training in speech pathology as well as speech therapy. He received his Ph.D. in 1934, held a research fellowship at Iowa for two years, then proceeded to Western Michigan University where he has been ever since. He resigned his administrative duties in 1966, and at that time was named a distinguished professor. ASHA cited him as an educator, therapist, researcher, author, and administrator who had earned worldwide recognition in various fields of speech correction.

Van Riper had a rough beginning for his Iowa years. This is another relatively minor incident but, like Bryngelson's, it helps indicate the state of affairs at the time. Very soon after Van Riper arrived in Iowa City, Travis was leaving for a week of lecturing throughout the state. "I'd just get in the car and drive from one place to the other," Travis explains, "lecturing every day, maybe two or three times a day, in one place and then going on to the next." Bryngelson suggested that the trip would give Van Riper a good chance to get acquainted with Travis, so Van Riper went along as the driver. Van Riper's stuttering was so severe at the time that he was practically speechless. Travis tells what that meant:

> We would go to a hotel and I would have to get our rooms. We would go to a restaurant and he would just nod when I ordered, take the same thing. On the road he wouldn't say a thing so I sang, the only song I knew, "There's a Tavern in the Town." I can remember saying when I came home that I had never been lonelier or more bored in my life! Well it was years later that he talked about it too. He said he thought he would go stark raving mad on that trip. He loathed the food I ordered. He couldn't stand my singing. He hated the song. So when he got home he went to work. He practiced saying every item of every menu he could remember. He said them out loud, over and over, when he was alone. When he could say those, he began on the song. He tackled it word by word, verse by endless verse, until finally he could bellow his way clear through—and on that day he figured he had it made! I wish you could hear him tell it!

Steer received his M.A. at Iowa in 1933 and his Ph.D. in 1938, then went to Purdue University where he has remained since and where he has distinguished himself as both a speech pathologist and psychologist. His work has centered in the laboratory (Travis calls it one of the most beautiful he has ever seen); his extensive writing has appeared in journals in the areas of speech pathology, audiology, voice science, military communications, instrumentation, and psychoacoustics.

Fairbanks came to Iowa as a speech major and took a prominent part in University Theater productions, but, after differences with Mabie, shifted into Psychology. He received the M.A. degree in 1934 and the Ph.D. in 1936, then taught voice and phonetics and a clinical course in voice and articulation disorders at Iowa until 1944, spending part of 1943 on wartime research duty before going into the army the following year. Following his army service he joined the faculty of the University of Southern California, and in 1948 moved to the University of Illinois (where one of his students was Jay Melrose, who received the Ph.D. degree in 1954 and joined the University of Iowa faculty in 1963). Fairbanks was on the staff of the Stanford Research Institute at the time of his death in 1964. He first published his widely used *Voice and Articulation Drillbook (4)* in 1937, when he was a member of the faculty at Iowa. He later gained unusual stature as a teacher and researcher in speech science, becoming widely known for his studies in delayed auditory feedback and for his servo-system theory of the speech and hearing mechanism. He was a leading figure in research in the science of electronic communication, where his particular interest was the study of speech in compressed and expanded forms. For this he devised instruments which held pitch constant while the words-per-minute rate was changed—instruments which have continued in use in research in this relatively new field. (See, for example, the special issue on speeded speech, *Journal of Communication,* September 1968.)

Morris, whose Ph.D. at Iowa was earned in 1936, went on to devote himself to special education and to administration in education. He was chairman of the Department of Speech and director of the Special Education clinics of Indiana State Teachers College from 1938 to 1946, was director of the Ohio State University Speech and Hearing Clinic the next two years, and in 1948 became president of Southern Illinois University.

Powers came to Iowa in the fall of 1935, a clinical psychologist with seven years of field experience. In her work she had become increasingly aware of the importance of speech in human behavior and of the great lack of both information about speech problems and procedures for dealing with them. She received her Ph.D. in 1938 (at the midyear convocation, when Steer also got his degree and when George Gallup, another Iowa great who had done innovative work with Seashore, was the speaker). She returned to Chicago, where she had been psychologist for the Institute for Juvenile Research, to take a position with the Chicago Board of Education as psychologist and speech pathologist in its Bureau of Child Study. She held that position for ten years, next became Supervisor of Speech Correction, then Director of the Division of Speech Correction, and in 1958 became Director of the Bureau of Physically Handicapped Children and Division of Speech Correction, a position she held until her retirement in 1968. Her Honors citation from the American Speech and Hearing Association lists among her contributions the organization and development "practically single-handedly" of the speech correction program in the Chicago public schools and her achievements, through lectures, workshops, conferences, and example, in bringing to educators in the public schools and in teacher training centers a sense of the importance of public school speech correction.

Koepp-Baker, who received his Ph.D. at the end of the 1938 academic year, was in 1968 professor emeritus of speech correction, pathology, and audiology at Southern Illinois University. He pioneered in work with organic speech disorders, particularly with cleft lip and palate, and in the area of the team approach to rehabilitation. His ASHA Honors citation refers to the fact that he was the first speech pathologist to be appointed to a full professorship in a major American medical school. His teaching career took him to a number of universities, including Iowa, Illinois, Pennsylvania State, Washington, Tennessee, Northwestern, Colorado, and Western Carolina College.

Hawk and *Simon,* predating Travis, made contributions that came to
figure importantly in the development of the Program at Iowa, and in a
larger sense in the development of the emerging discipline of speech
pathology and audiology. Hawk's commitment to the importance of speech
correction goes back to 1909 when she first began to try to help children
with speech problems. Her ASHA Honors citation includes these
sentences:

> In a large measure the place of speech correction in special education
> was insured by the mature and scientific manner in which she
> approached and developed the methodology of clinical speech. She
> wrote about speech disorders, and originated and described methods
> of treatment, when no journal represented the profession and there
> were no books of consequence in the field. As the first woman to be
> granted the Ph.D. [at Wisconsin in 1922] with major emphasis in
> speech, her insistence that training be basic and comprehensive
> encouraged universities and colleges to develop course programs in
> this area.

She taught for ten years at Mount Holyoke College, then engaged in
clinical work and teaching in California, and in 1966 became a consultant at
the School for the Visually Handicapped, Los Angeles.

Simon had graduated from Northwestern University before he came to
Iowa to study with Seashore. After receiving his Ph.D. at Iowa in 1925, he
returned to Northwestern and there proceeded to build that institution's
clinical and laboratory center and professional training program in speech
rehabilitation. For many years this amounted to a pioneering venture. He
became widely known as a lecturer and for his leadership in general speech
education. He did research in a number of areas and reported on this in
extensive writing for scientific journals. He became adjunct professor of
logopedics at the University of Wichita in 1966. He died in 1967.

Scholars and Stutterers. Both scholars and stutterers were numbered in the
"remarkable group" attracted by Travis' work. In some instances scholar
and stutterer were the same person. Two notable examples, Johnson and
Van Riper, have been named. Two others were John Knott and Spencer
Brown who, like Johnson and Van Riper, came for speech therapy, stayed
for Ph.D.s in the Program, and went on to positions of leadership.

In terms of first contact with the Program, *Knott* predates the other three.
In 1968 professor of psychiatry, head of the electroencephalography
program in psychiatry, and director of the EEG laboratory in the
University's Psychopathic Hospital, he came to Travis for help with his
speech when he was still in grade school and Travis was in his first
postdoctoral year. Knott's father, later to be general editor of the second
edition of *Webster's New International Dictionary,* was then on the University's
English faculty. When the family moved from Iowa City, Knott's contact

with the Travis Program was broken, to be renewed once in intervening years, and then a second time in 1934, when he returned as a student to finish his B.A. and to go on for a Ph.D. (1938) with Travis. His interests turned early to electrophysiological procedures. When Travis left, Knott took charge of laboratory work in that area "temporarily" and then remained in it for years, moving soon from East Hall to the Psychopathic Hospital area where he continued to have his office and laboratory.

Brown first came to Iowa City at Thanksgiving time in 1933, when he arranged to begin therapy in the clinic the following January. Once at the clinic, he became so interested in speech pathology that he enrolled for graduate work. He earned his M.A. in 1935, his Ph.D. in 1937, then went to Ohio State, then to Minnesota, where he earned his M.D. degree, served in the army, and came back to Iowa to teach two years, 1947-49. Then he returned to Minnesota for his residency in pediatrics. He went on to pursue a double career as pediatrician and speech pathologist, in private practice in Darien, Connecticut, and in clinical pediatrics at Yale.

Early Arrivals. Among those who (like Bryngelson, Knott, and Johnson) entered the Program early was *Joseph Tiffin,* who came from South Dakota to Iowa as a philosophy major but shifted to psychology when he became interested in the new scientific study of speech. He enrolled in 1927, received his M.A. in 1928, his Ph.D. in 1930, and taught experimental phonetics in the Iowa Department of Speech until 1937. Fairbanks, before becoming a faculty member, was Tiffin's assistant. Tiffin's later professional career has been identified with Purdue University. He made notable contributions in the area of industrial psychology, particularly in vision, where his orthorater, now commercially produced, is widely used to measure visual acuity.

Harold Fossler finished his Ph.D. in the Program in 1928; *Leo Fagan* followed in 1929. Fagan and *Yorke Herren* had both received the M.A. here in 1927. Herren turned to medicine and an outstanding career as a brain surgeon. Fagan, after his Ph.D., taught for a time in the Speech Department where Seashore's student, *Milton Metfessel,* was developing a laboratory and a laboratory course for speech majors. Metfessel, later of USC, left Iowa in 1929.

Elwood Murray and *George Kelly* finished their doctoral training in 1931. Murray is with the University of Denver and the Institute of General Semantics, Kelly taught first at Ohio State, then at Brandeis.

Bessie Rasmus (Petersen), a speech major, had joined Orton's mobile clinic staff as a speech specialist as soon as she had her B.A. in 1926, and had a faculty connection from then until her resignation in 1937. For her M.A. in 1930 she helped develop the Travis-Rasmus Speech Sound Discrimination Test *(15),* the first such test on record. For some time she was, in a sense, the Iowa Speech Clinic: she was the clinician, and her office was the clinic.

She maintained close contact with the emerging Program in Speech Pathology through her work as a faculty member in the Department of Speech. She married William J. Petersen, superintendent of the Iowa State Historical Society, and after her resignation from the Speech faculty she turned to activities associated with the Historical Society.

Scott Reger was taking the (then) two-year course in medicine at the University of West Virginia to obtain a more complete background for graduate work in psychology when Seashore lectured there on the psychology of music.[2] Reger, with an undergraduate major in psychology and a more than passing interest in music—he played clarinet in the University symphony—was interested, went to the lecture, and in 1929, with an Eastman Fellowship, enrolled at Iowa in the doctoral program in the psychology of music. He liked Seashore "immensely," admired him "greatly," but recalls *(10)* that he had to conclude that Seashore was

> possibly ahead of his time. Certainly he was an innovator. I don't recall his telling me how he happened to get interested in the psychology of music but he used to love to sing and he played and sang in church and even conducted a choir. He was that kind, you know, when he started singing in the choir, it was just a matter of time until he would be directing it.

It was in 1931, two years before he received his Ph.D., that Reger moved from the psychology of music to the psychology of otology to fill the position first held by Bunch. He has remained in that position from that day until his retirement.

Lois Cobb (Kluver), here for both undergraduate and graduate (M.A. 1931) work, became the first person to hold a joint appointment in the Department of Otolaryngology and Oral Surgery and the Psychological and Speech Clinic, and remembered *(7)* that "the interns on nose and throat were not ready for any speech pathology. Scott Reger was fully accepted but I had to 'assert my rights' and did so with the help of Drs. Travis and Lierle and Dean Seashore!" (Dr. Dean Lierle was successor to Dr. Dean as department head. Miss Cobb married Dr. Herman C. Kluver, who took his specialty training under Dr. Lierle. The Kluvers established their home in Fort Dodge where he was in private practice.)

Don Lewis, who retired from the faculty of the Department of Psychology in 1968, first came to the campus as a speech major for the summers of 1924 and 1925. He had already, as a teacher and more or less informally on his own, done a certain amount of clinical work with stutterers. He returned to Iowa in 1931 for his M.A. (1932) and Ph.D. (1933, a study in timbre), both in Psychology. Following a shift of interest from speech to psychoacoustics, he worked closely with Seashore and Tiffin. From that beginning period on throughout his academic career he maintained close contact with students in the Iowa Program, and later with the Iowa Department of Speech Pathology and Audiology. This contact was primarily through his work as director of the sound laboratory and his teaching in psychoacoustics, then in foundations of measurement, scaling, and quantitative methods.

His excellence as an "instrument man" was demonstrated early when he fabricated laboratory equipment to produce and vary the timbre of complex sounds, and when he did much of the design and actual building of the so-called "dead room" (E-6, East Hall, a sound-absorption room different from the older sound-proof room on the second floor, built to keep sound from coming into the room).

One of his widely recognized contributions to the discipline of speech pathology and audiology has been in scaling, in the initial instance in relation to severity of stuttering, when as a member of a Ph.D. committee chaired by Johnson he challenged *(8)* the design of the proposed study; that story comes later. A highly disciplined researcher, he also was an early challenger of the dominance theory of stuttering. That story, too, comes later.

James Egan, who went on to distinguish himself for his work in communication at Indiana University, and who later moved to the University of Washington, then to Texas, was an assistant in Lewis' sound laboratory. "My prize assistant," Lewis calls him.

Arnold Small worked in the Lewis sound laboratory. This was Arnold Small, Sr., then a candidate for the doctorate in Seashore's psychology of music program. After the Ph.D. he joined the faculty of the School of Music. He was an outstanding violinist, concertmaster of the University orchestra. (His son, Arnold Small, Jr., after the Ph.D. in psychology at the University of Wisconsin, returned to Iowa in 1958 with a joint appointment in the departments of Psychology and Speech Pathology and Audiology.)

Milton Cowan, in 1968 at Cornell University, where he distinguished himself in the field of linguistics, arrived at Iowa in 1934, actually on his way to the University of Wisconsin to do graduate work in linguistics. He was a German major. In Iowa City he had a talk with Seashore, decided to stay at Iowa, and received his Ph.D. in German the next year, after doing his laboratory work with Lewis (Tiffin was chairman of his committee). He taught at Iowa until 1940.

One estimate of the contribution of some of these people appears in a paragraph Seashore *(11,* p. 118) wrote in 1941:

> For thirty years the central interest in the psychological laboratory lay along the line of acoustics; laboratory equipment, subjects for investigation, and research personnel at first strongly represented this interest, with the psychology of music as the objective. This soon

demanded concentration of work upon basic approaches to the science of acoustics, and speech and psychology joined hands effectively. In this development, Lewis, Travis, Johnson, Tiffin, Reger, Fairbanks and Cowan have had the leading roles. It is now realized . . . that every aspect of such problems as sound treatment of rooms, the evaluation of elements of carrying power of the voice, phonetic problems, and the selection and training of talent can be approached experimentally. The general science of acoustics already offers a respectable body of scientific information and techniques of treatment which daily increases and extends the mastery of the art of vocal utterance.

In additional citations in this same writing Seashore (p. 112) suggests that Metfessel, Tiffin, Lewis, Fairbanks, and Cowan gave "pioneer leadership in the conduct of research" in the new scientific approach to speech; that "with the work of Metfessel came our development of photographic procedures to take the place of the graphic method followed by Merry," and that "this immediately led to great expansion and a variety of techniques, opening up new possibilities for ready and accurate measurement in speech and music." He goes on to say (p. 118), after again noting Metfessel's pioneering, that Fairbanks "has given great distinction to this course in phonetics by directing and publishing research. . . ." And he mentions, in his discussion of linguistics (p.119), that "Cowan and his associates are among the pioneers sponsoring this basic laboratory approach which gives linguistic science the distinction of being an experimental science in itself."

The EEG Group. Also among those present was a group particularly interested in Travis' electrophysiological research, and from this group has come an impressive amount of leadership in the area today. These leaders include Knott, mentioned above; *Herbert Jasper,* who went into medicine and neurophysiology after his Ph.D. with Travis, became a renowned specialist in studies of brain physiology, in 1968 was with The University of Montreal; *Kumar Bagchi,* who was at Michigan and has now retired; *D. B. Lindsley* who, after his Iowa Ph.D. in 1932, received an NRC fellowship, worked at Harvard, taught at Brown and Northwestern, then at UCLA; and *C. E. Henry,* of the Cleveland Clinic, who in 1962 was president of the American Electroencephalographic Society. That office has been held by Jasper, Lindsley, and Knott as well. Henry received his M.A. here in 1938 and his Ph.D. in 1940. Jasper founded and is a past editor of the *Journal of Electroencephalography.* In 1968 he, Knott, Lindsley, and Henry all were consulting editors on the staff of this journal. (Three years after the close of the period covered in the present history, the great pioneering contribution which Travis has made to electroencephalography was given recognition in a salute to him by the national assocation at its 1971 convention, when he was elected a Fellow of the American Electroencephalographic Society.)

The Busy Thirties. The tempo of the work increased and the enrollment increased during the late twenties and early thirties. Travis recalls *(14)* that he began to have eight or nine Ph.D. candidates every year. In the M.A. and Ph.D. theses listed in Johnson's "Bibliography of University of Iowa Studies through 1954" (in *Stuttering in Children and Adults,* University of Minnesota Press, 1955, pp. 447-463), roughly half of the total were written for degrees granted in the period from 1927 through 1938—that is, granted in the period when Travis officially headed the Iowa Program. The tally is a few more than half for the M.A.'s and a few less than half for the Ph.D.'s *Ernest Henrikson,* who succeeded Bryngelson at Minnesota, came in the early thirties, receiving his Ph.D. in the Program in 1932, and going on to a career in the new discipline even though he had originally come to Iowa because of his interest in Charles Woolbert's behavioristic approach to speech. Woolbert died within months of his arrival on campus. *Gladys Lynch,* an English major who became fascinated by the scientific approach to speech, shifted to the Program to do her doctoral work with Travis. After her Ph.D. in 1932, she taught at Winona State Teachers College, then returned to Iowa where, as a member of the faculty of the Speech Department, she taught speech science with both Fairbanks and Curtis. *John Black,* later of Ohio State, was here for the M.A. in 1930 and the Ph.D. in 1935.

The four M's were here: *Morris, Milisen, Morley, Moser.* Morris has been mentioned; Robert Milisen received his M.A. in 1933 and his Ph.D. in 1937 and has developed his program at Indiana University; Alonzo Morley, Ph.D. 1935, is at Brigham Young University; Henry Moser, Ph.D. 1936, is at Ohio State. *Joseph P. Kelly* received his Ph.D. in 1932, with a study in nasality; *Rolland Shackson* in 1934, with research on action potentials in stuttering.

Dorothy Davis Tuthill received her M.A. in 1936, but had not finished her Ph.D. before Travis left. She received that degree in 1939. *Curtis Tuthill,* who joined the faculty of George Washington University later, also received the Ph.D. in 1939. Travis sister, *Vera Travis (Rasmussen),* also was a student in the Program, and after her M.A. in 1934 taught in Racine, Wisconsin.

Charles Strother, who would be called upon to head the Psychological and Speech Clinic after Travis' departure, arrived on campus in 1933. He had chosen to come to Iowa to study with Travis rather than go to Vienna to study with Froeschels and Scripture because he admired Travis' work, and in addition was fascinated by the public debate Travis was carrying on with Robert West of Wisconsin in the journals of the day. Before he came to Iowa, Strother had already made up his mind that speech pathology was going to be a major discipline and that he wanted a career in it. He had even begun that career by introducing and teaching the University of Washington's first course in speech disorders, and by initiating clinical work in speech at that institution, even if only on a very small scale. After he received his Ph.D. at Iowa in 1935, he returned to Washington and there continued both the teaching and the clinical work he had begun before, establishing Washington's first speech and hearing clinic.

Jeanne Kellenberger (Smith), B.A. 1933, M.A. 1937, in 1968 an associate professor, and since 1953 on the staff of the Department of Otolaryngology and Maxillofacial Surgery, was here in the Travis years in the unusual role of undergraduate graduate student. As a sophomore she was taking experimental psychology and there, because of her ambidexterity, was "discovered" by Travis and Johnson as an interesting subject in the ongoing handedness experiments. Thus brought into contact with the Travis laboratory and the Johnson-Travis experiments, she soon changed her major to speech pathology, with Travis' permission, but also with his warning that she would be taking graduate courses as an undergraduate. *Florence Glassman* of Iowa City, now Mrs. J. Harold Saks of Great Neck, New York, did the same thing at the same time. From their junior year on, both were working primarily at the graduate level.

Smith, in her undergraduate-graduate years, worked full time with Dr. Lierle and did her M.A., supported by an Eastman grant, entirely in psychology—it was all in psychology because by then she had taken all the speech pathology courses! One Christmas vacation, to satisfy part of the requirements in a course in psychological testing, she administered psychological tests to the children at the Iowa Soldiers' and Sailors' Orphanage (later the Annie Wittenmyer Home). Her graduate work was directed by Dr. Lierle, Johnson, and Dr. Andrew Woods, then head of the Psychopathic Hospital.

Warren Gardner earned his Ph.D. here in 1936. In 1968 in private practice in Cleveland, and founder of the international organization of laryngectomees known as the Lost Cord Club, he had earlier pioneered in hearing testing in the Iowa public school system. He later continued this kind of work in both Indiana and Oregon. (Iowa's Dean Seashore, Dr. Dean Lierle, and Scott Reger were pioneers nationally as well as within the state in hearing conservation, as noted later.)

Jayne Shover, who later was to become director for the National Society for Crippled Children and Adults (after 1967 the NSCCA has been known as the National Easter Seal Society for Crippled Children and Adults), was among those present. She earned her M.A. here in 1936, basing her thesis on her study of bilingualism and stuttering in East Chicago schools. *Esther Glaspey (Ogdahl)* was here for an M.A. in 1933, stayed on to work in the clinic a year, then after teaching in Rochester, Minnesota, was brought to Indiana by Milisen, and worked on the staff of a mobile speech and hearing clinic under the direction of Gardner. Later she set up and directed a speech correction and speech improvement program in the Indianapolis schools, continuing in this work until her marriage in 1941. She now lives in Independence, Iowa. *Vivian Roe,* who had been at Iowa for a B.A. in 1936, followed her at Indiana and, with Milisen, proceeded to do research (the Roe-Milisen studies) which has become well known in the field.

Dorothy Sherman, who after her B.A. in 1931 had been teaching and coming back summers for graduate work, received her M.A. in 1938, taking part of her work with Travis, and doing her M.A. thesis under Johnson. Her speech courses were all in speech pathology, not general speech, and so it may be said that her M.A. was in speech pathology. The degree was granted by the Department of Speech. She was later to return to the campus and to become a member of the central faculty of the Department of Speech Pathology and Audiology.

Lloyd N. Fymbo gave an unusual twist to the interdisciplinary approach by working not only within the Iowa Program, that is, within the departments of Speech and Psychology, but also in the College of Dentistry. His M.A. thesis (1933) was a study of the relation of malocclusion to articulatory defective speech. His committee included J. Elon Rose and L. Bodine Higley of the College of Dentistry, Harry Barnes of the Department of Speech, Bessie Rasmus, and Lee Travis. (Higley appears later in the Iowa story, and so does the College of Dentistry.)

C. Esco Obermann, whose Ph.D. work (1938) was a psychophysiological study (effect on the Berger rhythm of mild affective states) directed by Travis, stayed on briefly in the Department of Psychology and then proceeded to develop a career in rehabilitation work, spending many years in the army. He returned to the University, to a faculty position in vocational rehabilitation, in 1966.

CLIMATE OF THE TRAVIS ERA

In their writings and their conversations, the people who were at Iowa to work with Travis tend to use such words as "splendid," and "exciting," and "stimulating," when they try to describe how it was. It was a demanding time, they say, a friendly time, a time of amazing innovation.

The new enterprise seemed so important that "no effort was quite enough. There was always the urge to do more, the fascination of exploring a little further." "We knew that we were working on something central in the life of a human being. We weren't just puttering around on the fringes." "We talked, long and seriously, evenings, and far into the night." "Everybody had a new theory every week."

Friendships formed were deep, lasting through the years. There was the time, for example, when Mrs. Bryngelson became seriously ill with trichinosis, contracted when she tasted pork for some Swedish Christmas sausage she was making as a special treat for her husband. Their son was 22 months old. The Travises pitched in to help. So did the others, especially Mildred Freburg (Berry). "I doubt if we ever would have made it without her," Bryngelson says. Although she was deep in her own graduate work and teaching, she planned her busy days so she could tote the little boy to and from preschool and in general make herself useful.

Travis and Seashore. Johnson liked to call Travis "the Chief," and did so with gusto and affection, as Travis remembers. This title even crept into the ASHA's Honors citation which Johnson was asked to write, and which ended with this paragraph: "The ties that bind these students and former students to the warm, vivacious, brilliant friend whom they call 'the chief' are indeed strong. By all who know his scientific and humanitarian works and their ever-enriching influence, he is highly esteemed."

Some students called the sandy-haired Travis "Duke Airedale," too. "Bryng is the one who started that," Travis recalls, "but Johnson always called me Chief." Travis was truly one of the early Big Men on Campus in that day. He drove a sports car. He dressed well. "He was almost flamboyant," Lewis says, recalling those times. "He was resented by many persons. But he was also very well liked. He was respected and loved by many."

Johnson, speaking at the ASHA convention in Columbus, November 1950, described Travis as a "great teacher." One of the reasons he is a great teacher, he continued, is that he "specialized in not specializing." Dorothy Sherman *(12)* regards Travis as a very brilliant lecturer. "He made us forget both the temperature and the drowsy time of day in his one o'clock class on the sunny side of East Hall through one whole fiendishly hot Iowa summer."

Travis was not stodgy in his lecturing—he sometimes appeared, for example, with the needle electrodes of his brainwave equipment stuck in his scalp. Fairbanks liked to do a takeoff on this, Mrs. Travis remembers. "He would have those things all hanging down from his head, and he would put on an act of how Lee would come in all wired for sound and start right in where he had left off the time before."

Seashore himself was a colorful figure, a man of great vitality, of dignified mien. He was tall, handsome, spare, an avid golfer who played well and regularly almost to the year of his death at eighty-three. He made a business of walking, swinging a cane briskly and with dash. He gave up that cane when he reached his seventies, explaining *(10)* to a friend, "I don't carry one any more. I was afraid people would think I had to." And he liked to read when he walked, often newspapers, and especially on his daily trips between his office and his home, the big red brick house at the corner of Johnson and Brown streets. When Dottie Klein (now Mrs. Robert Ray, wife of the University's Dean of the Division of Extension and University Services) was editor of the *Daily Iowan* she remembers well one icy day when Dean Seashore, striding along and reading his paper, slipped, fell, hardly moved the position of the paper in the process, finished the paragraph, got up, and went on, unruffled and still reading, as if nothing had happened. He had an amazing way of seeming always in control of the situation, even when sitting on the ice.

And he managed time for the thoughful, friendly act. In the beastly hot summer when Wendell Johnson was trying write his Ph.D. dissertation and the Johnsons were living right under the metal roof of the Iowa Apartments—top floor, southwest exposure—it was Seashore, Mrs. Johnson recalls, who offered help. He had a tent, he said, and there was a spot on his lawn to pitch it. As things worked out, the Johnsons were able to survive without the move, but they long cherished the expression of concern. And Bryng Bryngelson *(2)* likes to remember the many little chats he had with the Dean, in Swedish. "He liked to keep in practice."

Learning How to Learn. "The most interesting period of my life," is the way Cowan *(3)* describes his student days in the Travis era. "There is no question," he continues,

> about the quality of the teaching. It was excellent. But a large portion of the learning was done by discussion among graduate students. There was a very stimulating bunch of young people with diverse backgrounds. . . . Looking back on it now, I realize that this is the period in which I not only learned most of what I was to need for the rest of my life, but also learned how to go about learning what I needed to know. It was an exciting, stimulating atmosphere and all of the people I knew had a high order of enthusiasm and dedication to innovative research. Criticism was honest and sometimes ruthless. I look back on these . . . years at Iowa as my version of the "good old days."

Challenge of Doubt. Van Riper *(16)* feels that

> those were the most exciting years of my intellectual . . . life. . . . We were free to think, urged to speculate, but bound to defend any proposition we had formulated. And not just verbally. Put it to test. Set up your design. How can you disprove it? The multitude of projects all of us were engaged in was incredible. . . . All of us helped each other, took part in each other's research, and argued, argued, argued . . . We organized our own seminars, prepared hard for our presentations in them, and learned deeply. . . . Charles Strother gave one of the presentations and I still remember it as masterful . . . [I remember] one night down in the basement of Psycho when Dr. Travis and I got action currents from a grasshopper embryo, undifferentiated protoplasm, which made it impossible, but the

developed film showed them. And we talked all night and outlined a whole new theory of neurophysiology, his mind leaping far beyond mine, but accepting my checking doubts.

In Van Riper's opinion, "the secret ingredient of that fermentation period was the challenge of doubt. Doubt was demanded. . . . we were commanded to question all statements of belief."

Spirit of Pioneering. Powers *(9)* remembers the Travis era as a very exciting time to be at Iowa. She goes on to say,

I presume Iowa has continued to be exciting but probably it couldn't be quite as exciting as it was then because this was a brand new field. We were making tracks into the wilderness. There was a spirit of pioneering that was felt by everybody.

There was a great deal of interaction between the students and the faculty those days at Iowa. Almost all of the students were on scholarships and therefore had duties and for most of them this meant they were involved in teaching and I think you could characterize the setup as not having the hierarchical arrangement that you get in so many faculties. So there was a great deal of challenging each other's point of view and a great deal of freedom to experiment with things. And you might say that even the patients in the clinic were interacting with the students too, so that the students and the clients and the faculty had this sense of common purpose.

Reciprocity between Research and Service. Powers agrees that the predominant atmosphere was that of research.

But there was interest in the clinical, too. Travis had both, even though research was first with him in his Iowa years. But as the graduate students began going out into public school programs and coming back summers—people like Jayne Shover, and Dorothy Davis Tuthill later, and Esther Glaspey—they were not primarily interested in research. They were interested in service even then. I'm sure it was very significant in the success of the whole Iowa group as it went out into its own realms of application that there was a great deal of interaction between the research and the clinical. As I said one time—in fact in my ASHA presidential address—there was that reciprocity between research and service that is stimulating to both and very good for both, which is corrective of both, and productive of ideas in both. And I think this reciprocity was found perhaps uniquely at Iowa at that time.

I suppose the greatest contribution of the Travis-Iowa school was demonstration of the fact that communication as an aspect of human behavior could be studied scientifically. Before this it had all been pretty much by rule of thumb. There was very, very little that you could call scientific before that time. Travis saw the possibilities of the application of scientific methods he had learned in psychology. And I feel that the concepts of tabulating and measuring and trying to objectify and quantify observations carried over, for example, in many dissertations in general speech.

I was at Iowa because of my feeling that speech was so extremely important. I felt this from my experience as a clinical psychologist. This was kind of virgin territory. And these two facts put together made it a natural thing to want to get into: something important, where little work has been done.

Team Approach. Bryngelson *(2)* remembers the climate at Iowa in his graduate student days as one that was

conducive to nothing but good work. Travis was a scientist, but he was an artist too. So was Johnson. In each there was an amazing combination of science and art, just as in Einstein, for example, with his music and his science. And I think there was something about this many-faceted personality in Travis that made possible the beginnings of the team approach which I see as an Iowa idea from those days.

You see, Travis had an advantage in his medical setting at Iowa. I remember one time there was a psychiatrist there by the name of Dr. Eric Lindeman who questioned that there was anything organic about stuttering. He thought it was all a social maladjustment. Well Travis said, "I'm not saying for sure that what I find is it. But I think it would be interesting if you did a little research on it." So Dr. Lindeman did and I furnished the subjects and did some of the tabulating. And after a while this started a kind of a team, consultation, sort of thing because I remember meeting with Lindeman, Travis, and with some graduate students and Dr. William Malamud on many cases. They talked over various cases and of course Travis had had an excellent orientation in many areas. Yes, Travis was very free in letting anybody work on stutterers. They didn't have to do it the way he did.

Intellectual Ferment. Spencer Brown *(1)* remembers that in his Iowa days

morale among the graduate students was high. We felt we were in the best training center in the country. We were aware of gaps in our training, but we tried to correct these by reading and hard work. I was away for a year and when I came back Iowa was better than ever. There were more graduate students than before and they had come from all over the country.

I remember the Speech Pathology Program of that period as one of great intellectual ferment and feverish research activity. The Orton-Travis cerebral dominance theory was beginning to be questioned, first by Johnson and Knott. Travis at that time was unshaken in his confidence in his theory but he made no effort to interfere with discussions of it and would have supported my clinical testing of it if I had been able to devise an approach—I had tried, but finally gave it up and used another problem for my doctorate. We loved Travis' flair and enthusiasm. We were encouraged by Johnson's friendliness and almost unlimited generosity of his time and ideas. Iowa was a great place to be.

Golden Era. Travis himself looks back on the time as a "golden era," but, he continues, "I don't believe we had any idea we were making history. I think we just went from one thing to the next and found it all very exciting." Henrikson *(5)* agrees that there wasn't too much "looking down the vistas of the future, so to speak. But I had a feeling that the group was moving along. And it was moving dynamically, creatively."

REFERENCES

1. Spencer Brown, correspondence with author, March 24, 1968.

2. Bryng Bryngelson, taped conversation with author, Minneapolis, February 27, 1968.

3. Milton Cowan, correspondence with author, March 25, 1968.

4. Grant Fairbanks, *Voice and Articulation Drillbook* (New York: Harper, 1937, 1938, 1939, 1940; final revision 1960).

5. Ernest Henrikson, taped conversation with author, Minneapolis, February 27, 1968.

6. Wendell Johnson, "I Was a Despairing Stutterer," *Saturday Evening Post, 229,* January 1957, 26, 27, 72, 74.

7. Lois Cobb Kluver, correspondence with author, March 18, 1968.

8. Don Lewis, taped interview with author, Iowa City, October 1, 1969 (a repeat, in effect, of a conversation April 5, 1968 for which a proper recording had not been obtained).

9. Margaret Hall Powers, taped conversation with author, Chicago, March 26, 1968.

10. Scott Reger, taped conversation with author, Iowa City, April 3, 1968.

11. Carl E. Seashore, *Pioneering in Psychology* (Iowa City: University of Iowa Press, 1942).

12. Dorothy Sherman, conversations with author, April 1968.

13. Florence E. Teager, correspondence with author, March 19, 1968.

14. Lee Edward Travis (and Mrs. Travis) taped conversation with author, Los Angeles, February 8, 1968.

15. Lee Edward Travis and Bessie Rasmus (Petersen), "The Speech Sound Discrimination Ability of Cases with Functional Disorders of Articulation, *Quarterly Journal of Speech Education, 17,* April 1931, 217-226.

16. Charles Van Riper, correspondence with author, March 19, 1968.

NOTES

[1] In 1969 and again in 1972, that is, after the end of the period recounted here, five more Iowa names were added to the roster of recipients of Honors of the Association: in 1969, James F. Curtis, Frederic Darley, Scott Reger, and D. C. Spriestersbach; in 1972, Dorothy Sherman. All have the Ph.D. from Iowa. All have been or are now members of the Iowa faculty.

[2] Dover Publications has announced unabridged republication of the 1938 edition of Seashore's *Psychology of Music*. The Dover announcement in the fall of 1968 includes this text: "This well-known work . . . summarizes and evaluates practically everything that has been known about the psychology of music until the past few years. . . . It remains the standard survey of and introduction to this important field of study for psychologists, biologists, musicians and teachers."

5

THE TRAVIS PERIOD: 1927-1938

When he finished his postdoctoral training in 1927, a few days before his thirty-first birthday, Lee Travis acceded to three positions: associate professor of Psychology and Speech, psychologist to the Psychopathic Hospital, and director of the Psychological and Speech Clinic. His faculty rank, unusually high for an initial appointment, was given to meet an offer from Northwestern. A year later his rank was advanced to full professor, this time to meet an offer from the University of Michigan. Dean Carl E. Seashore, writing in 1941 (*18*, p. 132), explains that "we felt we could not afford to let him go in view of the service and equipment which had already been built up." But, he adds that Iowa's action in meeting the offer "has been amply justified by the resulting developments."

Some of these "resulting developments" are suggested by a comparison of Travis' titles in 1927 with those he carried in 1938, the year he moved from Iowa to the University of Southern California. By that latter date he was professor of Psychology and Speech, director of the Psychological and Speech Clinic, director of the Psychological Laboratories, and head of the Department of Psychology. Also by then he had completed a two-year term, 1935 and 1936, as the fourth president of the American Speech Correction Association, now the American Speech and Hearing Association.

OFFICIAL DATES

The dates 1927 and 1938 officially mark the Travis teaching years at Iowa even though they fall short by at least three years of including the period when, for all practical purposes, he headed the Program. However, since the year 1927, and not 1924, is set down in University records it takes its place with other beginning dates in the history of the Program, as well as in the Travis leadership at Iowa and the sequence of developments in the Seashore enterprise.

RESEARCH-PROFESSIONAL MODEL

Travis (*26*) feels that the model for the Iowa Program as he knew it can best be described as *research-professional*. He goes on to explain:

> The laboratory was for research. So was the clinic. In other words, the

speech pathology work at Iowa in my years was mainly experimental. The purpose was always to find out why. We were always looking at the person with the problem. He had a mystery. He had a secret. We tried to discover it. It might be in the psychological realm. It might be in the neurological realm. It might be a combination. The whole research thrust had its roots in those early days. The research thrust came from the beginning.

The work continued to be strongly interdepartmental even though in a relatively short time at the end of the twenties there were major administrative changes in all but one of the five departments most closely allied with the Program. That one, of course, was Psychology. Seashore continued there.

In 1926 Merry resigned as head of the Speech Department and Mabie succeeded him. In 1927 Dr. Orton resigned as director of the Psychopathic Hospital and Dr. Thomas Brennan succeeded him; in 1929 Dr. Brennan resigned and Dr. Andrew Woods succeeded him. In 1927 C. C. Bunch resigned as psychologist of otology; two or three graduate students, in turn, succeeded him, and in 1931 Reger succeeded them. In 1928 Dr. Dean resigned as head of the Department of Otolaryngology and Oral Surgery and Dr. Dean Lierle, who had trained under him, succeeded him. In 1928 Dr. Baldwin, director of the Child Welfare Research Station, died, and Stoddard succeeded him.

Travis says that after these several changes he worked perhaps more closely with Seashore and Mabie, the remaining members of his original committee, than with the newer people, but always felt that he was part of Psychology, Psychiatry, Speech, and Otolaryngology. Stoddard's role became increasingly supportive, a fact often alluded to in later years by Wendell Johnson.

Dr. Woods welcomed students from the Program into his classes, and continued until 1936 to accommodate the Travis laboratory in the Psychopathic Hospital. And in Otolaryngology and Oral Surgery Dr. Lierle and Reger proceeded to standardize and refine audiometric procedures, carrying forward the work begun by Dr. Dean and Bunch, and cooperating with the Program not only by bringing its students into their laboratories and lectures, but also by giving special classes for them. Reger for some years was "loaned" to the Program by Dr. Lierle to do this teaching.

CLINICS

To identify the clinics of this period is all but impossible because they were still a relatively tentative element in the sense that they depended on the yet young laboratory and the even younger classroom for their form and shape. The Psychological Clinic is a good example of this. This Clinic had been established in 1908. Now, at least on paper, it was part of the outpatient service of the Psychopathic Hospital. But, as Seashore explains (*18*, p. 140), it had

> a rich and varied but somewhat amorphous series of shifts in scope, organization, and growth. . . . In operating the clinic as a practical center of origins in clinical psychology, certain principles of administration and organization have given tone and character to the Iowa movement. . . . First the policy of allocating and integrating activities outside the department of psychology or the central clinic proper through various offices, departments, schools, and colleges. . . . This tended to mask and outshadow, and often ignore, the central clinic; but the fact is that it has led to operations of a vastly larger scale than could have been maintained in the clinic proper.

The expression "speech clinic" becomes particularly confusing. There was Seashore's Committee on the Speech Clinic. There was clinical work in the Speech Department which sometimes appeared in the University catalogue under the heading of Speech Clinic. There were also summer clinics sponsored by that department, one in 1926 directed by Miss Barrows, for example. There was clinical work in speech in relation to the sectioned fundamentals course.

In the June 1926 University *Bulletin* (see Chapter 4), Seashore wrote about "elaborate plans" for "the maintenance of practical speech clinics," then went on to fashion his prose in such a way that he seems to give the impression that these clinics were indeed realities at the time.

In Travis' case, although he was officially the director of the Psychological and Speech Clinic, such a clinic was just barely in existence. What was happening, as he explains (*25*), was that he was studying stuttering in his laboratory. Stutterers came in to serve as subjects in experiments, and when they were there, what could be done to help them was done. But of necessity this was limited. "So I was the clinic. The students were the staff. There were no other appointments."

As work went on, however, new ideas and understandings developed, and clinical activity tended to polarize around these. By the end of the Travis period the Program had an identifiable clinic which had borrowed a bit from other clinics here and there to become the Psychological and Speech Clinic, the direct ancestor of the Speech Clinic of the sixties.

IN THE TRAVIS LABORATORY

Travis continued to be greatly interested in his electrophysiological research and in the problem of stuttering, but did not limit himself to these areas. Several of the doctoral dissertations he directed were on animals, on rats principally, on the microphysiology of the nervous system of rats. Travis estimates he operated on perhaps a thousand rats in that lab.

> And we got into studying dogs. But I became a rat surgeon. I would take out pieces of brain. I would plant electrodes in the brain and all this type of thing.
>
> And then my interest ranged. For example, I asked [Dr. Henry] Prentiss in anatomy to call me immediately if somebody died. And so one day a call came. I went into the chest of the cadaver and put the tone in the trachea right about at the bifurcation where the two bronchi come out, about there. I pushed a tone up through his trachea, up through the vocal cords, and out through his mouth, and got a picture of the tone I had put in and a picture of the tone I got out. And I matched these two and published this is *Science*. This was a bizarre experiment, but you see I wanted to see what effect these speech structures, as nearly normal as I could get them, would have on tone.
>
> Then this went over into vowel theory. And I was interested in aphasia too. And of course in the mystery of stuttering. And especially in neurophysiology.

Much of the experimentation in his laboratory, first in developing the so-called Orton-Travis dominance theory *(24)*, then in supporting it, involved electrophysiological research, and from this came an interest in handedness since the dominance theory sought to explain stuttering on the basis of a difference in the cerebral dominance pattern between stutterers and nonstutterers. Electrodes were placed on given muscle masses or needle electrodes were stuck into the muscle mass on either side of the subject in order to measure the arrival time of the nerve impulse on each of the two sides.

HANDEDNESS RESEARCH

Another procedure was to change handedness and see what effect that might have. Stutterers would immobilize their dominant arm, usually with a cast. They used to do things like playing badminton outdoors with their "other" hand. At one time there were about thirty adult stutterers on the campus with arms in casts! One of these was Johnson. In fact, he was one of the first. Travis remembers him and Van Riper as his most enthusiastic and cooperative subjects: "I started with Johnson. And he was in everybody's doctoral dissertation. The breathing records were his. The voice records, the masseter action potential records were his. And I ran some knee-jerk experiments and he was in those. And he was the subject in blood chemistry. If he wasn't asked to serve as a subject he would volunteer."

The White Rat. Wendell Johnson had fun writing about this under the title of "My Experiences as a White Rat," a manuscript he began when he was a student, and revised several times but apparently never published. It is now with his papers in the University archives. In one of the later versions he explained, "I have served as a white rat in approximately one hundred and fifty experiments. . . . In the course of those . . . experiments I have had a white rat's view of several branches of science: general psychology, abnormal psychology, clinical psychology, educational psychology, psychoanalysis, speech pathology, neurology, physiology, and biochemistry. It seems to me that if one is to evaluate science in these fields, one must eventually go directly to the white rat."

A 1929 draft begins,

> I am probably the champion white rat in my part of the country. In other words, I am a laboratory subject. I am like a mechanical toy: press a button and I will do something. Again, I am like the Bible: students have proved almost everything by means of me. Men who work in laboratories have got almost everything out of me from a knee jerk to a tonsil, for it has been my curious job to contribute great quantities of first-hand evidence as to why we behave like human beings.
>
> Since I am a laboratory subject, naturally I observe with accumulative astonishment that among all the charming eulogies to the heroes of science there is not even a pamphlet to the memory of the chaps who take off their shirts to be jabbed. . . . Every time science advances a step, it leaves a scar on some white rat, four-legged or two.

He listed the chapters he planned to write: "I am psychoanalyzed, I breathe and speak and hold out my finger, I study my life history, I become left-handed—almost, I deliberately make mistakes, I relax, I am brainwaved, and hypnotized, I become extensionalized, my personality is tested, my IQ is determined, I am conditioned."

Van Riper *(27)* also remembers his days as a "guinea pig" in the laboratory, and the cast on his right arm, and the voluntary stuttering, and all the rest. "And cerebral dominance was in the air. No cult, either. It was something to test, an hypothesis." Van Riper was reminiscing about all this recently, speaking of the years of clinical experimentations and casework where he and Johnson, "as therapists, laid the foundations for our concepts of the nature and treatment of stuttering. Good talk; long talk; ideas!"Then he added, "We both made our way from the swamp of stuttering by our own struggle. Yet before us still was the mountain we must surmount before we could see the promised land—the ultimate conquest of that ancient disorder for all men. He took one route, I another, yet somehow it was very comforting to know that the other was climbing too. Then he died and ever since I have felt terribly alone."

A POINT OF VIEW

The foreward Travis wrote for Johnson's M.A. thesis (1929, "A stutterer's psychological study of his own case") amounts to a review of work in progress and suggests the spirit of questing and questioning that he encouraged. Down through the years the Program at Iowa has sometimes been criticized for putting too much emphasis on a given theory or project at a given time—and this can lead to endless discussions of how much is too much—and in view of that criticism it is interesting to note Travis' position here. Though he is writing during ascendancy of the dominance theory he does not take advantage of the situation to defend that theory. Instead, he sees the studies done as opening the way for other studies, he sees scientific research as search and more search. And in all this he notes that there is plenty of room for many points of view.

He writes:

For several years we have been carrying on in our Iowa Speech Clinic Laboratories [note that title] research in the field of speech pathology. We have utilized largely physical equipment to record the particular reactions we were studying. We have found that the stutterer presents definite functional neuromuscular derangements during stuttering and differs from the normal speaker in certain neuromuscular functions not directly related to speech. But we have not paid much attention to the so-called subjective or personal aspect of the stutterer's difficulty. He was not asked to tell us anything about his views of the organic disturbances which accompanied his speech efforts. The point is that we sought and secured strictly objective instrumental determinations of the various abnormalities.

It seems to us, however, that now we have gone far enough toward the solution of certain problems by the instrumental method to profitably take account of the subjective or personal side of the stutterer's speech disorder. Other workers have considered after a fashion this phase of the problem in securing introspective data from their subjects to serve as supplementary material at the time of experimentation. Our aim is somewhat different. We wish to secure the stutterer's statement of his own reactions to his stuttering organism and to society from the earliest incident of recall to the present moment.

We are very fortunate in having an ideal combination in Mr. Wendell Johnson, who is a stutterer with training in psychology and in writing. In addition he has served for three years as a subject in numerous objective studies of stuttering. It is in connection with this work that he has prepared his side of the story. In certain instances it supports the instrumental findings and completes the picture. In other instances it opens up new problems and suggests new lines of approach. One of the most obvious contributions involved in Mr. Johnson's study is its forceful opposition to many of the ridiculous theories held in certain quarters and its attack upon the neglect and misconception so characteristic of the popular attitude towards stutterers. Its chief value, probably, is to give parents and teachers an appreciation of the stutterer's real self—the feeling, sensing self which is so often ignored. Mr. Johnson's emphasis on the importance of this very point is not overdone. Our knowledge of the personal feelings of dozens of stutterers convinces us that he has expressed a common attitude among those with his type of disorder.

We wish to heartily recommend the value of the book [in book form it was called *Because I Stutter (7)*] as an original production for study by psychologists and psychiatrists; and we wish to emphasize its importance to parents and teachers who are concerned with the care of stuttering children. But over and above the contribution of this little book to psychology and speech pathology, it stands as a significant human document. In telling of the role that stuttering has played in his life, in the development of his personality, he touches on a theme that is of keen interest to the public generally. To a subject that has been strangely neglected—the place of the stutterer in a glib society—he has given the weight of vital interest and importance.

THE INTERMEDIATE PERIOD

An identifiable intermediate period in the Travis era began in 1929 and continued for about four years. In that time four major concurrent developments were initiated to the considerable advantage of the Program. These were: the move into larger quarters, and subsequent changes made possible by the additional space; the reorganization of the speech fundamentals course so that the number of research and clinical subjects was increased; the revitalization of the Dean-Bunch program in Otolaryngology; and the recording of brain waves in the Travis laboratory.

East Hall. The Program had been housed in the Travis area in the Psychopathic Hospital until 1929, in the Psychology and Speech areas in the Liberal Arts building (Schaeffer Hall), and in the Bunch area in Otology in the University Hospital. Included in the Psychology suite was the soundproof, lightproof, jarproof room, the building of which Seashore had supervised during his first summer in Iowa City.

In 1929, as Seashore (*18*, p. 29) tells it,

the psychological laboratory [by which it seems he means his department] had the great good fortune to join with education, philosophy, and child welfare in taking over the old central University Hospital which had some 300 rooms. This hospital had been standing idle for two years when one day I asked President Jessup what he was going to do with it. He said, "Well, that is an elephant on our hands," to which I replied, "Let us have it." He said, "All right," and I said, "Thank you, good morning," grabbed my hat and walked out to avoid the introduction of any qualifications. In about ten days Dean Packer [of the College of Education] and I took him a plan for the utilization of the building which was approved, I am sure, to the great advantage of the University as a whole. It was named East Hall because of its location on the campus.

The Travis unit remained at the Psychopathic Hospital, but for the rest the move began in the winter of 1929 and was completed so that some classes could be held in the new location by the beginning of the second semester. By the following fall everything was in operating order, and the building was dedicated in December 1930. At one point in the text of the dedication booklet there is mention of the cooperation between the Departments of Psychology and Speech, "especially in phonetics and speech pathology."

Speech pathology—that is, the emerging Program—was housed mainly on the ground floor of the east wing, and in third floor, center. Quarters were so spacious that every graduate assistant had an office. Seashore (*18,* pp. 136-7) says that when the "research laboratory for speech" was moved into East Hall from the Liberal Arts building "extensive space was allotted for a branch of the general psychological clinic with special emphasis upon speech disorders. This speech division was under the joint control of the departments of speech, child welfare, and psychology." This was the beginning of today's Speech Clinic, on a site it was to occupy for many years.

Fundamentals Course. Harry G. Barnes became full-time head of the Speech Department's fundamentals course (or "principles of speech," as it was sometimes called). The catalogue listing for the course describes it as "elementary speech training made specific to individual needs. The course is based upon diagnostic study of individual differences and abilities. . . . Opportunities of the Speech Clinic are available to students in the course." The purpose of the course *(4)* was "to correct or rehabilitate people's substandard speech, whether mild or extreme." (Barnes continued as head of the course until 1939 when he was succeeded by Franklin Knower who taught it until 1946.)

It was in Barnes's first year that the course was reorganized by Mabie, Travis, and Barnes. The purpose, as stated in the first issue of the *Archives of Speech,* in a footnote to an article by Elwood Murray and Joseph Tiffin, was "the segregation of students according to needs and disabilities and the building up of classroom and clinical procedures which are adapted to these individual needs." This article begins with this paragraph:

The recent reorganization of the required *Principles of Speech* at The University of Iowa, a course which each year enrolls nearly 1000 freshmen, has furnished an unparalleled source of material for the laboratory analysis of speech and voice. The first general survey of the freshman class revealed a surprising number of deficiencies in voice, articulation, enunciation and rhythm. While a number of drills are available for the improvement of these deficiencies, most of the available therapeutic measures do not seem to be based upon known basic differences between good and poor voices. Indeed, there seem to be very few data available on the nature of these basic differences.

Bessie Rasmus (Petersen) and Helene Blattner for some years did most of the clinical work with the fundamentals course students who had speech problems. Rasmus *(15)* explains that these students were rated on a seven-point speech performance scale, with *1* indicating a severe problem. She and Miss Blattner worked with those rated *1* to *3,* she taking the functional articulation cases, Miss Blattner, the voice problems. They used the Barrows auditory stimulation method. Their work was all in the Speech Department.

The course required a considerable staff. Many graduate students were employed, and several of these, over the years, became leaders in the Speech Pathology Program.

Psychology and Otolaryngology. Dr. Lierle *(13),* in his remarks as guest of honor of the American Otological Society in session in San Juan in 1966, suggested that "the origin of modern audiometric audiology is more closely associated with the name of Dean Carl E. Seashore than with any other individual," and that the triumvirate of Seashore, Dr. Dean, and Bunch "gave the initial impetus to what has developed into audiometric audiology as we know it today." He stopped short of mentioning the contributions which he and Reger, as successors to Dr. Dean and Bunch, made to audiology at the University, in the state, and in the nation.

Two of these contributions, closely related to the Iowa Program, had their beginnings in the intermediate period of the Travis years. The first is the offering of coursework to students in the Program. The second is leadership in public school hearing testing, which was new in Iowa but which in Seashore's career dated back to 1899, when he used his own audiometer for a series of such tests *(18,* p. 41).

These contributions appear to have been the vehicle by which Seashore's new psychology of otology (represented by Bunch, then Reger) came to join his new psychology of psychiatry (Travis) to produce the now traditional form of Iowa's Department of Speech Pathology and Audiology, in which speech problems and hearing problems are seen as integral parts of the larger central problem, which is human communication.

The study of hearing within the Program had for the most part been limited to the physiology of the ear in coursework on human anatomy. But as research increased in sophistication, and as associated clinical work grew, the importance of hearing problems in relation to speech became clear to Travis and his colleagues. Teachers who came back in the summers to continue their graduate work in speech pathology brought additional evidence, telling of the child who was not relating to his environment, who was withdrawn because he could not speak well because he could not hear well. Since Iowa-trained teachers had to go out of the state to work because there were practically no positions in their specialty within the state, and since many taught in Wisconsin's speech correction program, perhaps some sense of urgency in the expansion of the Iowa Program to include hearing testing was felt when Wisconsin passed legislation requiring its speech pathologists to have that training. At any rate, it is a matter of record that in the early thirties assistance was sought from Dr. Lierle and Reger. The request was for instruction in the techniques of hearing testing, and in the interpretation of test results. And all of this activity, let it be remembered, predated by more than a decade the coining of the word audiology and the general recognition of audiology as a science.

Reger *(17)* feels that when he arrived in Otolaryngology, still a graduate student, to continue on a part-time basis the work Bunch had begun, his credentials were not impressive. He had only his interest in music, his laboratory training in medicine and psychology, and a certain aptitude for building instruments. He had tested hearing with the Iowa pitch range audiometer in a course in experimental psychology, but he had no background whatever in the testing of hearing to localize the site of pathology in pathologic ears. So, he explains, "Dr. Lierle took me into a soundproof room one day and said, 'Now here's the way we do this, and that, and the other.' He walked out and that was my background in medical audiology. I hadn't done much work with tuning forks either and Dr. Lierle told me how to use them." And that was it. Reger frantically read stacks and stacks of books, and somehow he managed.

> I liked my work and seemed to get along and here I am. I've had only one job in my lifetime so you could say the labor turnover here has been zero.
> There wasn't a laboratory when I came over here. My first laboratory was in my office. Research money from the University was practically nil those days so with my own money I bought a drill press, and soldering irons, and this sort of thing because I wanted to build my own hi-fi and radios and so on. I've always built a lot of my equipment. I've never sent an audiometer back for repairs. I take care of it myself. And a lot of what I use here I build in my workshop at home.

In addition to his work with patients in otolaryngology, Reger tested the hearing of all University students, with the help of students from his class in audiometry. With his background in psychology he realized the desirability of using a standard procedure. There was none. So he devised, very early, a pulse-tone technique for obtaining threshold sensitivity, and used this in group testing with pure tones. "I think I was the first, possibly, to use that," he says. He and an audiometer designer and manufacturer, who saw him using it, patented it jointly.

As soon as he had his Ph.D. in 1933, Reger moved from part-time to full-time work in the department, was carried completely by the Otolaryngology budget, and began teaching and directing graduate work in the Program in Speech Pathology and Audiology through the regular year, and sometimes during the summer session as well.

Brain Waves. In the early thirties, probably 1931 or 1932, Travis, with Herren, and Dorsey, recorded brain waves from animals. John Knott *(11)* is convinced, on the basis of the best records he can find, that this was the first time this had been done by anyone in the midwest, and the third or fourth time by anyone anywhere in the United States. Travis sent a piece of the record to Seashore who at the time was vacationing in Whittier. Seashore wrote back, "Now what are you going to do?"

What he was going to do was already underway. In 1929 Hans Berger of Jena, Germany, had begun publishing about his work with human brain waves. Travis had learned about this and was fascinated with the idea of recording from humans, and had gone to work building equipment for this new purpose, particularly to investigate stuttering. Hunter by this time had been succeeded by Paul Griffith, another electrical engineer with a genius for instrumentation. As in the collaboration of Travis and Hunter, now the process went forward with Travis outlining the needs and Griffith building equipment to fill those needs. And, as before, the construction was done in the Travis Laboratory in Psychopathic Hospital. The first recording of human brain waves was made in the Iowa laboratories in July 1935.

Margaret Hall Powers *(16)* remembers that one of the first things Travis did was to run subjects. He saw he needed to run a lot of people—to be able to establish norms. "It was that new."

Travis and Griffith also made amplifiers for the University of Illinois, for Northwestern, and for Bradley Hospital in Providence. They shipped them to Chicago by freight train, and Griffith delivered the instruments, set them up, and gave instruction in their use. Griffith later went into electronics research with the signal corps of the army at Redbank, New Jersey, and appears in the Program for a second time in the fifties.

LABORATORIES IN EAST HALL

In 1934 a new soundproof room was built in the northeast corner of the ground floor of East Hall. A *Daily Iowan* item of May 24, 1934, refers to the construction as a room within another room, "a completely insulated cage . . . for use for experiments in music and speech." Seashore is quoted as saying, "Fundamental contributions to psychology are made when conditions can be controlled as in this sound-dead room."

John Black *(2)*, who was working on his Ph.D. at the time, recalls that Lewis and Joseph Tiffin "oversaw the construction of the dead room," and that, in addition,

> a lot of constructing was done. Tiffin tore up a piano to study the way the hammers hit the wires and to record this photographically [and thus built the Iowa piano-camera].
>
> Lewis was largely responsible for building the high speed string galvonometer oscilloscope that went with the dead room and the Henrici Analyzer. Lewis' work in reproducing sound wave form etched on glass discs was ingenious and pioneering. His later work with a homemade tone generator with variable phase was important in terms of the applications he made; an earlier model however had been constructed at Bell Telephone Laboratories.

Black sees these instruments and their building as examples of creativity in progress. And he mentions, as others have in these pages, that few instruments were purchased: "an oscillator, microphones, the Henrici Analyzer, and tools for the construction of other equipment."

The Henrici Analyzer. The Henrici Harmonic Analyzer was considered an exquisite machine. It cost several thousand dollars, and was one of only two or three in the country at the time. Tiffin *(22)* remembers it well. "In my early days at Iowa," he recalls,

> we were studying the sounds of speech and wanted very much to obtain an Henrici Harmonic Analyzer to analyze sound waves. The apparatus was manufactured by a Swiss company, and the Dean [Seashore] finally ordered one. Several months later it arrived. I will never forget our delight as we unpacked the "gadget." It came in a sealed lead box and, inside the lead box, the instrument was bolted to a hardwood frame. It was about 30 inches wide, 14 inches deep, and about a foot high. It was a precision made series of spherical integrators.
>
> To use it, you first had to enlarge the sound wave photographically so the wave length was (as I recall it) 40 centimeters. Then by carefully tracing the wave, you would find how much each of the first five harmonics contributed to its composition. Then you would change all of the gears, retrace the wave and find the contribution of the second five harmonics. By repeating the process many times, you would find the entire harmonic composition of the wave. It was a very time-consuming process, but we felt that with the Analyzer, we really were making great strides. Of course, the whole process of sound

wave analysis is now done electronically, much more accurately and in a fraction of the time then needed. But, at the time, we were certainly proud of the Henrici Harmonic Analyzer.

Travis *(25)* recalls that Fairbanks once did the incredible, made a harmonic analysis of a spastic's voice. "And," he added, gesturing to illustrate, "he found these terrific waves. It was amazing."

Move of the Travis Unit. In 1936 the Travis unit was moved out of the Psychopathic Hospital and into East Hall. Writing of this move, Seashore *(18,* p. 137) explains that, "since the psychological research done in the Psychopathic Hospital had concentrated largely on speech cases, Dr. Woods felt the experimental equipment built under the direction of Travis should be set up in the new joint laboratory in East Hall. When this was done the facilities for work in electrophysiology—much of which was of a fundamental nature pertaining to speech—were greatly increased."

The move involved not only the equipment built by Hunter and Griffith, but also many other items, for by then, Travis recalls, "we were buying equipment of Grass [Instrument Company]. And we moved all of this into the big area [north of the east-west hall, east wing, ground floor] up there. And we had it in that lovely soundproof room, lightproofed, electrically shielded and so forth."

With that move Travis became director of the psychological laboratories. He continued as director of the Psychological and Speech Clinic and, of course, as professor of Psychology and Speech.

In December 1936, soon after the laboratory was moved, Seashore wrote a memo to Dean Kay of the college of Liberal Arts (the memo is in University archives) requesting additional funds because the transfer of the "Travis Unit" had added considerable expense. He explained that the "psychology budget is carrying every expense for the experimental study of speech insofar as laboratory equipment is concerned . . . and is also carrying the [expense of the] psychological clinic, the speech clinic, and the reading clinic services. . . ."

THE CLINIC IN EAST HALL

Whether it was the Psychological Clinic and the Speech Clinic, as that memo seems to indicate, or the Psychological and Speech Clinic, as the lettering on the door proclaimed for many years, and as Travis and others remember, there was now a clinic in East Hall. This is the clinic that for a time was housed mainly in Bessie Rasmus *(15)* office on the ground floor of the east wing. It was also in Johnson's office. It was also found in other places, many recall, because before the situation became more structured the clinician and the client sometimes had to meet outdoors, or in the library, or wherever a convenient place could be found. Eventually, of course, all this changed.

As Powers *(16)* points out, however, this entire undertaking was still very new. And to have a clinic, however informal, was unusual.

> The cases came from all over. Many of them came in just for evaluation and diagnosis. And then we would try to work by sending written reports or guiding parents and working with local teachers or anyone who could do it, because there wasn't very much speech therapy going on. So it wasn't a very satisfactory operation because there couldn't be much follow up. There wasn't anyone professionally trained to follow up properly in carrying out speech therapy.

The work was mainly with articulation difficulties and the problem of stuttering. Relatively little was done with organic speech problems. Rasmus was in charge of most of the work in articulation, and Johnson was active in the work with stutterers, beginning his well-known *onset* studies *(9)* in 1934. A memo he wrote that year, now in the University archives, lists Charles Van Riper, Robert Milisen, Mack Steer, John Knott, Spencer Brown, Kumar Bagchi, and himself as "clinical assistants." Brown *(3)*, as one of those assistants, remembers the clinical activity with some misgivings. Like most of the students he was on a scholarship, for which he did clinical work two hours a day, five days a week. He was given a group of stutterers to work with and, he says, "I shudder at the thought that anyone with as little training as I should be given any clinical responsibilities. I got some—but not much—supervision, and it came in the form of conferences with Wendell [Johnson] and some of the other graduate student clinicians. But, he adds, "morale was high. We were aware of gaps in our training but we tried to correct these by reading and hard work."

In later years, Johnson would tell his classes of the ways therapy evolved. Then we would add, with a smile, that "it turns out we were doing many right things, for the wrong reasons."

> Mrs. Betty Walker *(29)*, remembering the years she spent as chief receptionist and general manager of the Clinic office in the early thirties, says that there was "very little to work with" then. Those were Depression days. So, in addition to the lack of literature, tests, clinical procedures, and all the rest, there was a lack of such mundane items as files and general office supplies. "But we managed," she adds. "We managed to set up a file system and take care of our patients as they came in and find places for those to stay who came from a distance. And the students took over as clinicians . . . and most of them are still working in the speech correction field."

Then she continues with this vignette of how it was:

> Dr. Travis asked me to take over the Clinic office in the south end of the east wing of East Hall in the spring of 1933. I had worked part

time there and in Dr. Travis' office in Psychopathic Hospital starting in the fall of 1931—spending mornings in the hospital and afternoons in the Clinic.

Dr. Johnson was a very bad stutterer at that time. He would come to the hospital and would read to me while I typed. Then we would usually walk back to the Clinic together. Paul Griffith also worked both places and the three of us would carry on as much conversation as possible along the way. Paul also was a very bad stutterer in those days.

One has many wonderful experiences during a lifetime. But my years with Dr. Johnson and Dr. Travis have been some of my most precious.

THE CURRICULUM

Students who were on campus during the Travis years remember that the formal curriculum within the Program was very limited, and that the heart of it was what was commonly referred to as Travis' introductory course. Travis' presentation in this course has been called "disorganized" by some, "wide ranging and challenging" by others, "stimulating" by most. "It opened many doors," they say. He more or less built the course as he went because there was practically nothing to work from. There was no literature to turn to. There was scarcely even a language for definitive discussion of speech and hearing problems; this too had to be devised as the work went along. But from the beginning he stressed the centrality of communication, and therefore its overwhelming importance in human behavior.

By the early thirties coursework included, as Powers remembers, Travis' course, Tiffin's and Fairbanks's course in experimental phonetics, Rasmus' in phonetics, Reger's in audiometric technique, and Johnson's in stuttering.

One way to fill the gap in formal course work was through those famous seminars. Reger recalls those the students themselves organized.

These were quite a thing. Someone would be appointed to talk about a certain subject. This was known in advance and of course Travis attended these, and Johnson, and Joe Tiffin, and Fairbanks, and Lewis, some of the sharpest people around here. And when you were to present a talk or paper you really worked at it. We'd get together at seven. We would have a formal presentation, then we would have coffee and cookies maybe, then we would talk till midnight—this was serious discussion.

Three or four days before one meeting I remember in particular an edition of the magazine called *Science* came out. Lots of people sent short articles in there to get priority for an idea or to present something new. Well Weaver and Bray had an article in there in which they had measured what they thought were auditory nerve action potentials up to 3000 to 5000 cycles per second. Now that is impossible with an ordinary nerve because of limitations imposed by the absolute refractory phase. So it looked as if the Helmholtz theory of hearing was not longer tenable, if this were correct. And if it were correct it meant that the auditory nerve was a special nerve which could do things and had capabilities that other nerves, so far as we know, did not possess. It also meant that the telephone types of theories of hearing were tenable, or some variation of this. So all we could do was sit there and talk about that.

Well later on we found out that this Weaver-Bray phenomenon was something different from what they assumed it to be, that when the ear responds to sound the cochlea generates an analog of the acoustic wave—an electrical signal which can be picked up from the round window. Also, in addition to this, there are auditory nerve action currents. But Weaver and Bray thought that they were picking up only auditory nerve action currents. And we sat up most of the night talking about it.

Powers recalls that each faculty member would have a seminar too.

And these were especially interesting because the instructor would go on in almost any direction the people wanted to go. I remember one of the most interesting seminars we ever had was one that Travis gave in psychophysiology. And everybody attended this, faculty and graduate students. And each one of us took a topic to really dig into and report on and I chose some of the aspects of vision because I knew less about that. Travis was trying to cover all the sensory processes, you see, as a basis for understanding the speech process and the hearing process much more thoroughly.

Course Listings. A list of courses taught by Travis appears for the first time in the University catalogue for the academic year 1924-25, when his name is given with the Psychology but not the Speech faculty, and his course is in "the clinical psychology of speech, a critical practical survey of the theories of speech pathology with clinical practice; designed as a fundamental course for those who are to practice or teach speech correction." The course is listed in both Psychology and Speech. In addition, in Speech, Giles Gray is listed for a course in the theory of speech and Barrows for classes concerned with the "application of phonetics to speech correction."

Reflecting Merry's pioneering in speech science, a "speech correction" listing of some kind had been carried in the catalogue by the Speech Department for several years. In the 1922-23 catalogue, for example, Merry is listed for a course in "the theory of speech; voice science and laboratory," and Blattner for one in "the correction of speech disorders." In that same year Fletcher appears in the Psychology listing for a "seminar in the psychology of corrective speech." In 1923-24 the Speech listing shows a "speech correction" unit, with the notation that the offering is being made "with the cooperation of the Child Welfare Research Station and other departments and colleges"; within the Speech Department this coursework is given by Barrows and Mabie.

From 1924-25 on through Travis' years at Iowa each catalogue carries his course in both Speech and Psychology listings. That year other coursework within the Program was given by Metfessel.

More or less the same pattern continues through the Travis years, with some of these names dropping out, others being added. Barrows, Bryngelson, Merry, Baldwin, Woolbert, Gray, for example, dropped out; Tiffin, Fairbanks, Fagan, Cowan, Barnes, Murray, Lewis, Johnson, were added.

Clinic Listings. In the 1928-29 catalogue, as since 1925, a "speech clinic" is included in Speech, this time with this descriptive paragraph: "Speech and voice disorders are handled in the speech clinic. Each individual case is examined, diagnosed, and treated under expert guidance. Such work offers exceptional opportunities for the student to come in direct contact with the research and clinical aspects of speech pathology. The clinic has on its staff speech experts, psychologists, social workers, and a psychiatrist, and the cooperation of the various departments of medicine."

Beginning with the 1926-27 catalogue, the Psychological Clinic is carried in the Psychology listing. The related course, taught by Travis, is described as "an introduction to the study of defective, delinquent, and unadjusted individuals."

In the 1929-30 catalogue, in a descriptive section on laboratories, a "Clinic in Speech Pathology" and the "Psychological Clinic" are listed separately. In 1930-31, the course listing shows this same separation, or distinction, whichever it may be. The note there is to the effect that "the psychological clinic and the clinic in speech pathology" are "located in two divisions": in the Psychopathic Hospital and East Hall. The former would be Travis', the latter Johnson's and Rasmus'.

General Semantics. When Johnson was named to the faculty in 1937, his courses were called "language and speech disorders," and "speech hygiene." In both of these he incorporated the tenets of general semantics, to which he had been introduced the year before by Count Alfred Korzybski's *Science and Sanity,* and Korzybski's insitute in Chicago. From this time onward, through his entire academic career, Johnson brought coursework in general semantics to his students, and used a general semantics orientation in his counseling activities, public lectures, and writing. (Johnson also encouraged his students to attend the Korzybski seminars. Jeanne Smith [21] recalls being there when Travis, Tiffin, and Fairbanks were among those present.)

STUTTERING THEORY

Stuttering theory was being developed in combination with the electrophysiological work of the period. Laboratory results in the dominance studies were always encouraging, but the clinical results never were, Travis recalled recently.

> We still find that the relationships between the two hemispheres of stutterers differ from the same relationships of nonstutterers. We have always found some evidence of disturbed cerebral dominance in stutterers. But I still don't know what to do about them. I maintained my interest in the possibility of cerebral dominance until I came to USC. At USC I had a big clinic and almost no laboratory so I did much more clinical work than at Iowa. And I had to get results. So I began to shift from this neurological thinking and approach to psychological. I picked out the modified psychoanalytical treatment as probably the best concept to work with and teach with. We began to look at stuttering more as a psychological than a physiological thing.

In Travis' years at Iowa, the dominance theory of stuttering came in for its first great public challenge in the mid-thirties. The word "public" is important in that sentence, because Lewis had challenged the theory as early as the fall of 1931, soon after he returned to Iowa for his graduate work, but it did not become a public challenge. He had planned a piece of research before he came here, then had proceeded with it at once after he arrived. "The results that I obtained," he says *(12)* "in what I thought was a critical study, were never published. Dr. Seashore refused to permit me to publish the results because they were contrary to the dominance theory."

It was four or five years later that Knott and Johnson began actively to question the theory. In 1936 they published an article, "The Moment of Stuttering" *(10)*, which Knott *(11)* suggests represented a break from the physiological point of view. This new approach was also used in another study, "A Systematic Approach to the Psychology of Stuttering," which the authors wrote about the same time, submitted for publication, and then recalled. It was finally published in 1955, in *Stuttering in Children and Adults,* where the two studies *(8,* p. 14) are described as developing "considerably" the "original notion," which was that

> the practical requirements of investigation would seem to be better served by dispensing with the arbitrary designation of some segment of the series of events in a moment of stuttering as *the* "stuttering." What would appear preferable to this is the adequate observation and description of the stuttering moment as a functional unit, together with determination of the variables related to it. Or, one may meaningfully investigate the functional relationships among the

various discernible parts or segments within the moment of stuttering.

Another basic study in stuttering theory, which also was written about that time but first published in this same book (chapter 8), was Van Riper's investigation of adaptation. Authors are Van Riper and Catherine J. Hull (Iowa B.A. 1931), who became Mrs. Van Riper, and who went on for her M.A. degree at the University of Minnesota when the two moved there.

As Knott remembers it, Van Riper was working on his theories at one end of the hall down in the clinic area of East Hall, and "Johnson and I were working at the other end of the hall. And some of our theories were slightly overlapping but at the same time not identical, and some were incompatible in terms of the treatment of the stutterer."

The three would try out each other's ideas, and eventually Johnson and Knott, as the latter explains, were working on

> an analysis of stuttering which essentially was that stuttering was the attempt to avoid stuttering, the well known paradox which has been in the literature and which has been carried on to this time. I was at that point intrigued with the psychological problem of attention and so we wrote another paper in which we tried to bring out the problems of the stutterer in attending to certain cues in the speech environment. And this led to a string of studies. Johnson noticed that if you reread material repeatedly, you tended to stutter in the same places. That was what we called the consistency effect. We began to develop experiments around this then.
>
> Actually Van Riper got the initial adaptation effects and when we started to study adaptation we discovered consistency. Then we came to the matter that you could predict. Of course, we were already at this one anyway in our analysis of our own speech. We were going around carrying small notebooks and writing down everything we observed about our own speech at this time. And we came to the conclusion that we could predict precisely where we were going to stutter. So we ran our experiments on this. This was a new kind of experimentation, or at any rate nobody else had been doing it.
>
> At this point we sort of broke with Travis. I can remember I was the one who was elected to present our concepts to Travis' class. This, of course, was a very stressful situation. He invited us in, you see, to present our material. And of course we came out with a flat, almost a complete, rejection of the dominance theory. Travis was clearly troubled by it, but the kind of being troubled that you understand. He had a heavy investment in his own theories. There was never any personal reaction, however. We used to argue with him, and it was all out in the open. It was actually quite stimulating because he would try to reduce our approach, you see, would try to raise all of the arguments against it, when he could marshal evidence against it. It was all done, you know, across the table.
>
> When we made that original presentation to his class we still left in

the possibility that there might be some neurophysiological defect which led to minor speech hesitancy. I don't know when we gave up the neurological area entirely. You know, it's just irrelevant, probably not very important, except maybe in unusual cases. I'm still [1968] inclined to believe that there may be some cases that are not stuttering, as we think of it generally, which give symptoms which tend to resemble those we call stuttering. I have some personal reservations on this.

Knott did an EEG study with stutterers for his master's thesis. Little difference was found between stutterers and nonstutterers, or between stutterers when they were speaking and stuttering and stutterers when they were speaking and not stuttering. He goes on to say:

> this was another one of the reasons why I was moving away from any sort of neural theory. We had one stutterer that gave some odd effects that I would not call artifacts. Travis and Malamud wrote this up and made something out of it. Travis and I did another paper in about '36 or 7, a somewhat more adequate study. And, again, we were unable to get any differences between stutterers and nonstutterers.

> I kept at this problem after Travis left and had one Ph.D. candidate who did some other ways of treating data which seemed to show that there might be a statistical tendency for the left half of the brain to be a little different from the right half of the brain in normals and a little less different in stutterers. We were able to confirm this in another study done by a master's student, once we knew what we were looking at specifically. But this is, again, a statistical trend and not one that I feel has any clinical relevance to the problem as we know it. Actually, now that we have more adequate kinds of ways of treating data with computers this thing simply ought to be redone some time.

Johnson and Knott did many studies together in the thirties, continuing their collaborative thinking and research through 1938, when Knott received his Ph.D. and moved into electroencephalography, while Johnson remained in speech pathology. The more they worked on their new idea, the more central the avoidance concept became; that is, they began to view stuttering as something that the speaker does in trying not to stutter. They tried out procedures to implement the idea clinically. One was "the bounce" (*8*, p. 219, No. 4), which was probably originally Bryng Bryngelson's brain-child. It required that the speaker repeat as easily and effortlessly as possible the sound or syllable on which he expected to have trouble.

"This meant," Knott explains,

> that the stutterer would try to stutter in a more relaxed manner and that carried inherent in its own execution what we came to call

voluntary stuttering because, if you're going to do this and do it well, you must become a devoted and purposeful stutterer. The interesting point was that the minute that Johnson and I became purposeful stutterers we stopped stuttering. We had nothing more to avoid. I usually worked with one or two stutterers who were in the clinic, and it was amazing the rapid degree of relief that could be produced by simply putting people out on a schedule where they called telephone numbers, went to stated places, in real life situations, where they were to stutter on purpose.

I remember talking to Johnson perhaps within a year of the time he died [1965], about the treatment problem and about the basic philosophy of stuttering. We agreed that actually, except for refinements, much of the groundwork had been laid down then in that analysis of ours on the moment of stuttering. It's been refined, there've been changes, there've been new ideas brought in to sort of bolster it but [in that analysis of ours] there was a complete rejection of the neurological point of view as a meaningful component.

IOWA AND THE SCHOOLS

During the thirties, the Iowa Program produced a fair share of M.A. degrees for people interested in them as preparation for teaching. But few of these prospective teachers stayed in the state because there were almost no public-school positions in speech correction in Iowa. So it was that for several years many Iowa M.A.s went principally to schools in Wisconsin, Pennsylvania, New York, and California to work as speech correctionists. Dorothy Sherman (20) described the situation in a lecture to a class in the Department of Speech Pathology and Audiology at Iowa many years later, telling how scarce clinical speech positions were in Iowa in 1938, the year she received her M.A. degree. She recalled knowing of only one school system in Iowa in which attention was then being given to speech correction; that was in Des Moines.

Before this, she had been teaching in Faribault, Minnesota, where she was offered a position as speech clinician to begin September 1937. Instead, taking Travis' advice, she accepted a position as classroom teacher in the Des Moines system. She worked on her M.A. thesis while she was teaching, and received the degree the following summer. She continued to teach in Des Moines and had been in junior high school work there for nine years before there was finally an opening so that she could move into speech correction. So it was not until 1946 that she entered the field professionally.

That first year in speech correction in Des Moines was memorable, however, because of her assignment. She was charged with developing a program and a plan for the city, and for that year she was given carte blanche—she had no obligation as to case load, number of schools covered, calls made, and so on.

In the fall of 1946 Sherman applied for and received Iowa certification for public school work in speech correction. Hers was the first such certificate to be issued in the state of Iowa. Her service as classroom teacher stood her in good stead because in those days certification required not only training in speech correction, but also experience as a classroom teacher. She continued another two years in the Des Moines system, in speech correction, before returning to the University to go on with her graduate work.

In the thirties Seashore, Travis, Paul Packer of the College of Education, and others developed within the Iowa Program a schedule of courses to train graduates at the M.A. level for professional work in the field. So The University of Iowa became a leader in training speech correctionists even while Iowa as a state lagged in using them.

Iowa Public School Hearing Testing. Reger became involved in the earliest part of what eventually became Iowa's statewide hearing testing of school children. Some suggest that this hearing testing may have helped move the state toward a speech correction program.

A school principal wrote to Seashore in 1933 or 1934 to see if someone could come out from the University to do hearing tests. "You see," Reger explains,

Dean Seashore had sent people out to try his measures of musical talent, to standardize them, in school systems, and so was known. But this really is amusing because this principal had an ax to grind. I got permission from Dr. Lierle to be gone two or three days, I load the stuff in my car, and I drive up there and I meet this man and I soon find out that he thinks his son is hard of hearing. So that was his motivation, or at least it was part of it! I don't know how truly interested he was. Anyhow, I tested the school children and found a few with hearing problems.

Then the word got noised about that the University would send people out to do hearing tests. I went to a few other places. But there were too many requests coming in, I couldn't leave my job here to do this. Then Dean Seashore called me in and said we were going to need a full-time man, and who would this be, and I don't remember details now, but Warren Gardner was the man. That was in 1936.

I talked with Warren and demonstrated and we checked the calibration of the earphones to see if they always put out the same intensity when the same electrical signal was going into them. I took him down to Davenport. I worked with him there a day or two and saw things were moving smoothly and came back home and he stayed there and tested the hearing of every school child in Davenport. Well then he travelled around over the whole state. It was a full-time job.

Seashore (*18*, p. 41) said he thought that Iowa's was "the first state undertaking of the kind. The project was made entirely self-sustaining in that superintendents who wished to have their pupils examined could invite Dr. Gardner for such time as was necessary on the payment of a moderate sum per diem."

There were quite special administrative problems involved. "It is interesting to find," Seashore said,

> that for very good reasons the department of otology in the State University Hospital could not sponsor this movement because it would immediately have been interpreted as proselytizing for patients. Not even the extension division, representing the board of education, dared to sponsor the subject for the same reason. Nor did we feel safe in designating the service as official from the psychological clinic. To get around these difficulties, I simply issued a bulletin to city superintendents of the state describing the necessity for the work, the methods of procedure, and some of its significant features, purely as a personal note, introducing the specialist in this field who had been trained for this work in our laboratories but who could not be regarded as a member of our staff. This is a rather striking example of how careful the University has to be about treading upon the area of professional services.
>
> It is also a striking example of the necessity of educating a profession to a new point of view. When Dr. Gardner came into the field, his first step was to call upon the school physician and other physicians who might be interested, explaining his services would neither prescribe nor treat but he would expect the cases discovered to be referred to physicians. So far as I have been able to learn, no objection to this procedure was raised by any physician throughout this experiment.
>
> It is also interesting to note that after three years of operation, the state board of education passed a rule that this service should be discontinued, apparently on the ground that too many cases of imperfect hearing would be discovered in the schools. But the edict came too late; the experiment had already served its purpose, and the schools are now [1941] introducing audiometry with their own instruments and on their own initiative.

PUBLICATIONS AND PUBLIC RELATIONS

The school hearing testing program was one of several ways in which Iowa's new Program was becoming known widely within the state and considerably beyond its borders. Travis and his associates, notably Johnson, made it a point to attend meetings of teachers and parents around the state. So did Seashore. University publications (the 1926 summer session bulletin cited above, for example) carried the message of the new work.

Much the same can be said of those issues of *Psychological Monographs* which were edited by Travis and Tiffin during the same period. The *Monograph* publications grew out of the series known as the *University of Iowa Studies in Psychology*, which Seashore and G.T.W. Patrick had started in 1897. Patrick edited the first three volumes of the *Iowa Studies*, Seashore went on from there until 1927, then Christian Ruckmick of the Psychology Department faculty became editor.

Psychological Monographs. Later Seashore moved away from University production of a publication of this kind or like the *Archives* series and instead, with graduate college funds, bought entire *Monograph* issues from the *Psychological Review*, using these publications to carry the Iowa studies (see, for example, volume 36 of the *Psychological Monographs*, which includes studies by Seashore, Travis, Metfessel, Simon, and Mildred Davis, and which lists, on page 263, the studies in the Iowa series). Many studies from within the Program became the text for the series of *Child Welfare Bulletins* which the University began issuing in the early days of the Station.

When the American Speech Correction Assocation (now ASHA) began to publish the *Journal of Speech Disorders* in 1936, people from the Iowa Program used it extensively. The first issue (March 1936), for example, carried a study by Travis, Tuttle, and Cowan on heart rate during stuttering. And in the same issue a bibliography of studies from 1933 to 1936 in speech, voice, and hearing disorders began, to continue through succeeding issues. It was compiled by Iowa's Morris, Ohio State's Russell, and Syracuse's Heltman from the speech clinics of the three institutions, "through the interest of the directors," Travis, Russell, and Heltman. Iowa studies show prominently in this listing. A year later Johnson and Knott, with others, published a seven-part series on the psychology of stuttering.

Books that came out of the Program in this period included Travis' *Speech Pathology (24)*, Fairbanks's *Voice and Articulation Drillbook (5)*, Johnson's *Because I Stutter (7)*, and Van Riper's *Speech Correction (28)*. Books by those closely associated with the Program included Seashore's *Psychology of Music (19)*, Orton's *Reading, Writing and Speech Problems in Children (14)*, Gray's *The Bases of Speech (6)*, Barrows' (and Cordts') *The Teacher's Book of Phonetics (1)*, and *Speech Sounds of Young Children (30)*, by Wellman and others of the Child Welfare Research Station staff.

A series of programs known as the Speech Clinics of the Air was inaugurated over the University station, WSUI, in 1935, and numerous articles appeared in the daily papers.

Scholarly Journal Publications. In the academic community the contact was made primarily through a vigorous publications program in a variety of professional journals. As Travis explains,

the majority of the studies we did regularly and as theses were published. We seldom had anything turned down and I don't believe I ever did, but we must remember that we had advantages then that we don't have now. In the first place this was a new field. And in the second place there was room in the journals then.

I published an average of seven or eight studies of my own every year through that period. These would appear in the *Archives of Neurology and Psychiatry, Journal of Experimental Psychology, Journal of General Psychology, American Journal of Physiology, Science, Quarterly Journal of Speech,* all these journals, medical journals, psychology journals, speech journals.

Archives of Speech. The publication called *Archives of Speech* was a University of Iowa journal which Seashore (*18,* p.35) described as emanating from the Psychological Laboratory under the editorship of the Department of Speech. It was founded by Mabie, and five issues appeared between 1934 and 1937, when it ended. One issue was on debate and was edited by Craig Baird who recently retired from the Iowa Speech Department. Of the four other issues, two were on experimental phonetics, edited by Tiffin, and the other two were on speech pathology, edited by Travis. These four amount to something of an overview of the research being done those years within the emerging Program.

THE END OF AN ERA

The Travis era ended just as it began, in a period of great change. In 1937, when Travis had been in his new duties as director of the Psychological Laboratory about a year, Seashore retired at the age of seventy-one, forty years after he had joined the University faculty, thirty-two years after he became head of the Psychology Department.

Travis, now forty-one and a faculty member for ten years, succeeded him. Travis moved into the Seashore office just inside the front entrance of East Hall; for a year he administered from this office. In 1938 he resigned, shaken by internal difficulties not in the Program, but in another area in the Department. He joined the faculty of the University of Southern California where Metfessel was head of the Psychology Department. As at Iowa, Travis had a joint appointment in Psychology and Speech, and again was director of the Psychological and Speech Clinic. He interrupted his USC teaching for four years of service during World War II (lieutenant colonel, Army Air Corps), after which he returned to USC and continued in the joint appointment. For two years he headed both the Speech Department and the reorganized Speech and Hearing Clinic. In 1957 he joined the Gilbralter Savings and Loan Association as vice-president in charge of personnel and public relations. After three years in that position he went into private practice in Beverly Hills, and in 1965 became dean of the graduate school of psychology of Fuller Theological Seminary. He has continued his laboratory research, has continued to find brainwave differences between stutterers and nonstutterers, continues to wonder what those differences mean, and has been intrigued to note that others are searching and wondering too.[1] One of his major later writing projects was the field's classic *Handbook of Speech Pathology (26)* which he edited, and to which he contributed as an author. The book was published in 1957 and revised by Travis, a decade later.

In the perspective of history, a Travis *(23)* article of 1936, called "A Point of View in Speech Correction," appears as a sturdy bridge between his administration at Iowa and those to follow. "The primary concern of speech correction," he wrote, "is the person." And then he develops that idea in a way which anticipates much of the thinking and writing which was to come in the Iowa Program in later years:

> ... speech correction considers primarily the individual. As the individual acts as a whole, so does he talk. . . . Speech is the joint by which the speaker articulates with the person spoken to. . . . Speech joins his world within and his world without. . . . In order to understand the individual's speech, it is necessary not only to understand his speech organs, but his person as a whole. . . . It is essential that the speech pathologist, above everyone else, should be a thoroughgoing student of the whole person.

REFERENCES

1. Sarah T. Barrows and Anna D. Cordts, *The Teacher's Handbook of Phonetics* (New York: Ginn & Company, 1926).

2. John Black, correspondence with author, March 26, 1968.

3. Spencer Brown, correspondence with author, March 24, 1968.

4. Paul Wilson Davee, "Definition of the Philosophy Underlying the Recognition and Teaching of Theater as a Fine Art in the Liberal Arts and Graduate Curricula at the State University of Iowa," Ph.D. dissertation, University of Iowa, 1950.

5. Grant Fairbanks, *Voice and Articulation Drillbook* (New York: Harper, 1937, revised 1938, 1939, 1940, and 1960).

6. Giles Wilkeson Gray and Claude Merton, *The Bases of Speech* (New York: Harper, 1934, revised 1946).

7. Wendell Johnson, *Because I Stutter* (New York: Appleton, 1930; out of print and now available, microfilm or xerography, on special order from University Microfilms, Ann Arbor, Michigan, 48106).

8. Wendell Johnson, *Stuttering in Children and Adults* (Minneapolis: University of Minnesota Press, 1955).

9. Wendell Johnson and associates, *The Onset of Stuttering* (Minneapolis: University of Minnesota Press, 1959).

10. Wendell Johnson and John R. Knott, "The Moment of Stuttering," *Journal of Genetic Psychology, 48,* 1936, 475-480.

11. John R. Knott, taped conversation with author, Iowa City, May 29, 1968, and conversation with Dr. Paul Huston, Iowa City, June 1973.

12. Don Lewis, taped interview with author, Iowa City, October 1, 1969.

13. Dean Lierle (with Scott Reger), "The Origin and Development of Audiometric Audiology at the University of Iowa," *Transactions of the American Otological Society, 54,* 1966, 19-23.

14. Samuel T. Orton, *Reading, Writing and Speech Problems in Children* (New York: Norton, 1937).

15. Bessie Rasmus Petersen, conversation with author, Iowa City, April 10, 1968.

16. Margaret Hall Powers, taped conversation with author, Chicago, March 26, 1968.

17. Scott Reger, taped conversation with author, Iowa City, April 3, 1968.

18. Carl E. Seashore, *Pioneering in Psychology* (Iowa City: University of Iowa Press, 1942).

19. Carl Emil Seashore, *Psychology of Music* (New York: McGraw-Hill, 1937; reissued, New York: Dover Publications, 1968).

20. Dorothy Sherman, classroom lecture, Introduction to Speech Pathology and Audiology, University of Iowa, 1962, and conversations with author, 1968-72.

21. Jeanne Kellenberger Smith, correspondence and conversations with author, January-February 1972.

22. Joseph Tiffin, correspondence with author, April 1, 1968.

23. Lee Edward Travis, "A Point of View in Speech Correction," *Quarterly Journal of Speech, 22,* 1936, 57-61.

24. Lee Edward Travis, *Speech Pathology* (New York: D. Appleton-Century, 1931).

25. Lee Edward Travis, taped conversation with author, Los Angeles, February 8, 1968.

26. Lee Edward Travis (Ed.), *Handbook of Speech Pathology* (New York: Appleton-Century-Crofts, 1957).

27. Charles Van Riper, correspondence with author, March 19, 1968.

28. Charles Van Riper, *Speech Correction* (Englewood Cliffs, N.J.: Prentice-Hall, 1939, 4th ed., 1963).

29. Betty Walker (Mrs. G. A.), correspondence with author, March 20, 1968.

30. Beth Wellman and others, *Speech Sounds of Young Children* (Iowa City: University of Iowa Press, 1931).

NOTE

[1] For example, F.K.W. Curry and H. H. Gregory, "The Performance of Stutterers on Dichotic Listening Tasks Thought to Reflect Cerebral Dominance," *Journal of Speech and Hearing Research,* 1969, 12, 73-82; and R. K. Jones, "Observations on Stammering after Localized Cerebral Injury," *Journal of Neurology, Neurosurgery, and Psychiatry,* 1966, *29,* 192-195.

6

THE STROTHER PERIOD: 1939-1947

In 1939, four years after he had received his Ph.D. under Lee Travis, and about a year after Travis's resignation, Charles Strother returned to the University to become director of the Psychological and Speech Clinic in East Hall, and in that capacity to head the Iowa Program in Speech Pathology. He succeeded Travis in both positions, becoming the second director of that Clinic and the second head of the Iowa Program.

His eight year administration, spanning the national emergency of World War II, was deeply involved with the problems which the war generated at the University and throughout the academic community—problems that were related to short staff, increased enrollment, accelerated coursework, unusually heavy workloads, crisis planning, and, in general, responses to unprecedented demands.

Strother's own responsibilities were in both speech pathology and clinical psychology. In speech pathology, he was particularly concerned with the area of functional speech disorders. In clinical psychology, his work contributed to pioneering activity which led to increased definition of that emerging discipline. During the years of his leadership there came to be a gradual separation of speech pathology from clinical psychology, a maturing of speech pathology, and its initial linking with audiology, another emerging discipline.

This was the situation at Iowa, but it is to be understood as part of a national development as well. At both levels it reflected the stimulating effect which mobilization seemed to produce. And it reflected, too, the fact that speech pathology was in its third and fourth generations, and was neither unique to Iowa nor isolated there.

There are those who suggest that clinical psychology and audiology became distinct entities sooner, and that speech pathology matured more rapidly, than they might have if there had been no war that required this extraordinary growth spurt. All three disciplines were drawn into the heart of the crisis early because all three could be expected to be helpful in rehabilitation of the casualties that the war so soon produced.

Immediately after he received his degree, Strother had gone back to the University of Washington, where he had taught before, to establish a clinical program in speech and hearing disorders. When he took up his new duties at Iowa, he had the advantage of four years of experience behind him.

His administration at Iowa began after a major disruption in the Program in Speech Pathology: "When Travis departed there was a great deal of uncertainty as to what would happen because he was clearly the leading figure in the Program. And this uncertainty," Strother found *(19)*, "affected both the staff and the student populations.

> Then this had hardly begun to settle down when the war started. And this, again, was a period of great disruption. Many people on the staff left. The people who remained were exceedingly busy.
> The Clinic in East Hall was growing. And at the same time it was changing character because an increasing proportion of the cases there were concerned with problems other than those related to speech.
> Then my duties were increased so that I had responsibility for clinical psychology in the University Hospitals, that is, in the Psychopathic and General and Children's Hospitals. And that work led to the beginning development of a training program in clinical psychology there.
> The University, very soon after this, was assigned an Army Specialized Training Program project in counseling psychology. I was involved in this. Later this project led to a further increase in the faculty workload when many of the individuals who had come originally for the ASTP training returned for graduate work in clinical psychology.

Bette Rae Bartell (Spriestersbach), a graduate student at the time and later a clinical associate (Iowa M.A. 1945) in the Department of Speech Pathology and Audiology, recalls *(18)* that Strother's classes seldom held to a permanent meeting place. More often than not they went where he happened to be working as classtime. That was one way of managing as his increasingly heavy duties moved him about the campus.

Growth and Separation. Strother explains that, "with the development of a more formal program in clinical psychology, the distinction between graduate training in clinical psychology and in speech pathology and audiology became sharper. It was inevitable that the two programs should become distinct entities, rather than being combined as closely and informally as they were during Dr. Travis' period."

There were indeed many differences between the Strother and the Travis periods. The pioneering aspect of the work, the singleness of purpose, the smallness of the group, even the difficulties of depression years, all tended to draw people together in the Travis period. But the first flush of pioneering now was gone, and so was the singleness of purpose because new areas opened up and new opportunities developed. The group was no longer small, it was larger and growing steadily. The depression had changed to the wartime boom, and the war itself became a divisive influence in terms of the demands it made on faculty. Beyond all this, the central purposes of the two administrators were different. To Travis the research thrust was central, while Strother had a commitment to the search for the best and most effective use of the yield of the research. Both men remembered and honored in their work the original laboratory-classroom-clinic progression outlined by Seashore; but their priorities, perhaps by both necessity and choice, were different. The laboratory had come first in the Travis period. Now a new sense of the importance of the clinical enterprise was taking shape.

Appointments. Strother's appointment at Iowa was at the rank of associate professor in the Departments of Psychology and Speech, and officially director of the Psychological and Speech Clinic. That directorship was one of three positions left open when Travis resigned. The other two were head of the Department of Psychology, and Director of the Psychological Laboratories. John Knott accepted responsibility for the electrophysiological segment of the laboratory, moving into that work very soon after Travis left. John McGeoch became head of Psychology but, like Strother, did not come to Iowa until 1939. George Stoddard was interim acting head of Psychology. Strother's colleagues within the Program were Wendell Johnson, Grant Fairbanks, and Scott Reger who continued to be "loaned" by Otolaryngology.

As director, Strother had primary responsibility for the Psychological and Speech Clinic but beyond that, as far as the clinical area was concerned, his role and the roles of Johnson and Fairbanks were not at first defined. Within a short time, however, the three men divided responsibilities: Johnson worked with stuttering, Fairbanks worked with the voice and articulation disorders, and Strother took over organic disorders of speech and also what could be called the Psychological Clinic, that is, the cases involving problems other than speech. Thus all the developmental and behavioral problems—retardation, for example—came in his province. The Clinic, as it had since 1930, remained on the ground floor in the east wing of East Hall. It was "both the Speech Clinic and the Psychological Clinic, operating as one," Strother points out. And it remained so for as long as he was at Iowa.

In this period a regular outpatient clinic was held every week in East Hall, with Strother responsible for the scheduling of cases that came into the clinic, for the procedures that were used in evaluation, and for chairing the staffing at the end of the evaluation. "And this common intake continued," he explains, "but after we began to divide the cases the others developed their own staffing. My staffing was primarily for the cases in organic disorders or in psychology."

CLINICAL PROCEDURE

At the beginning of this second period of the Program, soon after Strother arrived, he and Johnson and Fairbanks revised all of the clinic records, the case history forms, the diagnostic procedures that were routinely used, and the procedure for staffing the cases. He feels that a significant contribution to diagnostic procedure in the Psychological Clinic was made by Sidney Bijou, a doctoral candidate who had come from Wayne County Training School and had had a good deal of clinical experience before he entered upon his degree program. After Bijou received his Ph.D. here in 1941, he was at the University of Washington for twenty years, then became professor of Psychology and director of the Child Behavior Laboratory at the University of Illinois. In 1961 he was awarded a senior fellowship by the National Institute of Mental Health.

ORGANIC DISORDERS

In Strother's graduate years at Iowa there had been little work in organic disorders of speech, and few organic problems were brought to the clinic. He saw only one or two cleft palate cases and no celebral palsy in that training period. But in his years as administrator there was a great deal of interest in organic problems. Some of Strother's students, for example, went to dentistry and anatomy for further training.

There was work beginning on the design and use of obturators in cleft palate. There was a great deal more sophistication in aphasia and in cerebral palsy. I think what had happened was that as speech clinics began to be established, these cases just came in at Iowa as at other places. And so you had to learn about them and you became interested in them. This was certainly my experience. When I started in the clinic at the University of Washington, my training had been principally in stuttering and articulation disorders. But people with organic disorders, aphasia, and so on, began to come in. And you had to accept them and assume responsibility for them, and so you had to learn fairly quickly. And this broadened out into a more basic understanding of these disorders.

INTERDISCIPLINARY APPROACH

This broadening reinforces interdisciplinary activity. I think one can't overstress the importance of the interdisciplinary atmosphere at Iowa, both when I came there as a student and when I came back as a member of the faculty. All through the history of the Iowa Program it's been, I think, an exceedingly fruitful influence. And I attribute a great deal of it to Seashore. He succeeded in demonstrating how effective it could be, and this just opened doors all over.

As head of the Department of Speech, which increasingly was becoming the home of the Iowa Program, E. C. Mabie was developing a relationship with the Program that was in many respects like Seashore's in an earlier time. Strother recalls that in one of his first

conferences with Mabie when I came back [I saw] another facet of that very complex man. He was anxious to stimulate his staff to advancement. He was interested in moving into new areas. And so when I was first on the staff he offered me a great deal of free time if I were interested in taking a degree in medicine. And he had in fact talked with the Dean and really paved the way for me to enter the medical school and take a medical degree. And I started. I took some courses but the more I looked at the curriculum the more I felt that most of it was not relevant to my interests and I didn't want to continue. And I guess Spencer Brown was the only person who went ahead and took a degree in medicine.

The interdisciplinary cooperation in this second period of the Program was, in Strother's opinion, "very stimulating and very fruitful and quite unusual for that time. It is not to be found in many places even now."

Psychiatry. Among cooperating disciplines was psychiatry, he adds.

Quite a number of the students were doing their theses in the laboratories at the Psychopathic Hospital. This was, as a matter of fact, an important gathering place for students. And Dr. Malamud and Dr. Lindeman, in particular, were very generous in offering courses, and students were free to sit in on seminars and case discussions. And so this was an important area. I think that it's fair to say there were probably three centers: Psychopathic Hospital, Otolaryngology, and East Hall, where the students congregated and around which the work, both formal and informal, developed. And from those three centers there was development in both the investigative program and the clinical aspects of speech and psychology.

Child Development. The Research Station joined in the effort, he recalls.

There was another influence that was quite important, and that was in child development, in the Child Welfare Research Station. I had a good deal of contact with the students in child development and the staff in that area. And this, I think, was an important contribution to many of the students who had particular interest in this area. Robert Sears and Kurt Lewin attracted a large following of graduate students and many of the students in speech pathology took courses in Child Welfare.

Otolaryngology. Another cooperating discipline was otolaryngology. Strother says:

> I remember particularly Dr. Lierle's willingness to spend time with students from Speech and from Psychology, and to offer seminars for them, to work with them on research projects. And the students studied with Scott Reger. Then his work, of course, had a great deal of influence on the development of audiology as a profession.

CHANGES

It seems remarkable that there would be this strong interdisciplinary cooperation, given the major changes in administrative personnel which, war or no war, affected the Program in important ways. Stoddard resigned in 1942 to become Commissioner of Education of the state of New York. Sears succeeded him as director of the Child Welfare Research Station. Dean Carl E. Seashore came out of retirement to take over the Stoddard duties as dean of the Graduate College. And within the same year McGeoch died and was succeeded as head of the Department of Psychology by Kenneth Spence. This was an interesting new trio of leaders: Seashore, Sears, and Spence.

Seashore's official duties did not relate to the Program as closely now as they had in the pioneering days when he also was head of Psychology. He found the time, however, and the energy too, to know and be known by those in it. His critical appraisal of work in progress was no less keen than before, it seems, and he was no less willing than he had been before he retired to make suggestions and to give encouragement. His creative genius was still very much alive.

In terms of both history and inclination, Spence and Sears did not have the same kind of interest in the Program that Seashore had. And as each of the two new men sought to strengthen the work in his own area, these areas tended to draw away from each other, and Psychology tended to draw away from the Program as well. Beyond this, an acknowledged philosophical difference between Spence and Sears became a force of some magnitude, Strother observed, when Kurt Lewin joined the Station staff.

As time went on, and as the graduate training in clinical psychology developed, the Program gradually migrated almost completely, in terms of administration and budget, out of Psychology and the Child Welfare Research Station and into the Department of Speech. It continued to enjoy warm and relatively unchanged relationships with Otolaryngology and Psychiatry. Staff appointments reflected the situation. Johnson, for example, whose support had been carried by Child Welfare, Psychology, and Speech, was taken off the Child Welfare budget entirely, and his support from Psychology was greatly reduced when he was named a full professor in 1945. Most of his salary then came from the Speech Department budget.

Other faculty changes had a direct bearing on the Program. Dewey Stuit joined the Psychology Department faculty in 1939 and was, by himself, the staff of its reading clinic. Franklin Knower succeeded Barnes in 1940 as head of the Fundamentals course. That same year Orvis Irwin, whose interest was children's speech development, joined the faculty of the Station. In 1943 Gladys Lynch was named to the Speech Department faculty to teach in the speech science area. Her Iowa Ph.D. of 1932 had been directed by Joseph Tiffin. Jacqueline Keaster taught hearing conservation classes in the 1943 and 1944 summer sessions. In the fall of 1945, after a year in audiology in the armed forces, working with Fairbanks in the Army Rehabilitation Program at Borden General Hospital, she became a regular faculty member at Iowa with a joint appointment in Otolaryngology and Speech.

Though they could hardly be called faculty changes, two assistantship appointments of the period, both in Speech, are of interest in view of the later careers of those concerned. The appointees were James Curtis and D. C. Spriestersbach.

JOHNSON'S INNOVATIONS

The academic year 1939-40 saw two innovations by Johnson: one was his course in general semantics, the other the Demosthenes Club. The general semantics course is said *(4)* to be the first offered in any university under that title. Except for one year when he was on leave from the campus, he continued to teach this course one semester each academic year from 1939 until 1964, the year before his death. In 1939 the enrollment was twenty-three, the next year it was twenty-seven, the following year, thirty-five. By 1947 it was 148 and stayed over one hundred from then on. The course was also offered by correspondence beginning in 1951, and was broadcast by station WSUI during the fall semesters of 1956 and 1959. The course was always within the Program of Speech Pathology and Audiology but drew its enrollment from the total University—as Johnson put it, "from Art to Zoology."

In the spring of 1940, Johnson started a new group for stutterers in which he used the general semantics approach. It was called the Demosthenes Club. Through the Club people with a stuttering problem came together, discussed their problem, helped each other as much as they could, and made an effort to talk in all kinds of situations, to strangers as well as friends. Among other things, they gave programs for various organizations with the dual purpose of working on their speech and helping their listeners to understand the problem of stuttering. Eventually other Demosthenes clubs were formed around the country by Iowa students as they went out. (This was the beginning of the Speech Correction Fund, sponsored jointly by the National Society for Crippled Children and Adults and the American Speech and Hearing Association.)

An additional activity for Johnson in these years was participation in a Works Progress Administration (WPA) survey of public school speech and hearing services in Woodbury, Cass, Polk, Dubuque, and Scott counties. Stoddard was director; Johnson, technical director. As a part of his work, Johnson wrote the report, published in August 1942, pointing out that of the 30,000 school children surveyed "a considerable number" needed help with speech and hearing problems. Remedial instruction was given at various sites for 173 children who had been found to have "speech and reading deficiencies." (John Chotlos, a doctoral candidate, analyzed the survey data and developed his dissertation from them. He received his Ph.D. degree in 1942.)

A NEW CONSTELLATION

In a period coinciding almost exactly with the time span of the Strother administration, Don Lewis of the Psychology faculty undertook a series of studies in his department which were to lay the foundation for a constellation of research in the psychological scaling of severity of speech disorders. The impetus for his studies came from within the Program and the resulting research fed back first into the Program, then into the Department, and on into the larger field of the discipline of speech pathology and audiology. Research in the area has continued at Iowa ever since.

The story of the beginnings of the innovative enterprise reveals something of the times and the climate and the people at Iowa, as well as the nature of the research itself. Lewis recalls that this country was going into military conflict, but that the United States was not yet directly involved as a combatant. Then, he continues *(11)*, "I was asked to do some work on possible effects of high level noise, and vibrations, on the efficiency of pilots operating planes. The project was financed by the National Research Council through their Pilots Committee and I had half a dozen people working on it." These included Earl Schubert, later on the faculty of the Iowa Program, and I. E. Farber, later on the faculty of the Department of Psychology.

For his project, Lewis "borrowed" the shelter house on the riverbank just north of the University theater, a shelter built for skaters, swimmers, and canoeists, and later used as a laundry room by students living in nearby barracks. He borrowed it from E. E. Harper, director of the Iowa Memorial Union and head of the School of Fine Arts,

much to the distress of Harper and others. They thought this high-level noise would disturb everybody on the west side of the river. But we got the room anyway and it was ideal for the purpose. It was a stone building.

We set up operations there, got loud speakers that would produce 120 dB level noise, set them up on a platform. We could induce enough vibrations to make your cheeks rattle and we could measure the level of the vibration with a meter that we put on top of the skull. And we measured perceptual motor skills too with what we called a Mashburn apparatus (Col. Mashburn of the Air Force had designed such an instrument) which we built. It was a six-channel device and you moved it in connection with a wobble stick in a certain one of the channels depending on the appearance of lights on the stimulus panel.

Well, it was quite an elaborate setup and we went on for most of two years. We took many kinds of measures. We found it necessary to have not just gross categories or gross periods of time but to know what had happened after a certain onset.

I was more or less imbued with this whole notion at the time of a committee meeting for a doctoral candidate by the name of Leigh Carroll Douglas, an older man who had been on the staff at Grinnell College. The research plan followed the technique that had been used over and over, of comparing the brain waves of a group of so-called stutterers with those of a group of so-called normal speakers to see if they differed in any characteristic way.

Measuring the Severity of Stuttering.

At that time, as I recall, there had been attempts to get at severity of stuttering in two ways. One was to make a count of moments of stuttering over a given period of time or a given amount of material. Occasionally the speech would be recorded, on the old acetate discs, in my laboratory. But more often the clinician would just listen to the speaker and mark on a copy of the material when instances of stuttering occurred. The other method was to use Brown's five-point scale. [See Spencer F. Brown, "Loci of Stutterings in the Speech Sequence," *Journal of Speech Disorders,* 1945, *10:* 181-192.]

At this committee meeting I raised a ruckus. I asked why, if they were going to take brainwave records, why they didn't take measures that would let them know when the stutterer was indeed stuttering. Johnson himself had emphasized that oftentimes the stutterer doesn't stutter. Johnson himself could demonstrate this. By this time, after 10 years around here, he had become more or less expert at speaking. He still stuttered but he had brought himself to the point where he would tend to have some control.

Anyway, that was my thesis: Why don't you take a recording of the speech along with the recording of the brainwaves and get some measure of the severity of the stuttering at the time that the brainwave record is taken. Well, this went for the preliminary meeting and then we had another meeting and I said essentially the same thing. Johnson, blushing and stuttering very badly, said, "DDDDon Lewis, if you think you can mmmmmeasure the severity of stuttering, dddddamn it, why dddddon't you ddddo it!" That was the challenge. So that was the start.

Lewis outlined a plan and one of his doctoral candidates, Margaret Lee Dassler, began the research with him, recording the speech of fourteen stutterers reading material of three levels of difficulty. The researchers then dubbed out nine-second segments, because that length could be managed easily in terms of the number of revolutions on the old disc recorder: "We could control that better than the timing because the 33 rpm record went around so many times and that was a nine-second length." So Miss Dassler did some ratings of these segments and then went off, abandoning her Ph.D. program, to marry William Lichty who was teaching at Southern Methodist.

Next came William Grings, who had been a student at Dubuque, then doing graduate work at Iowa, and who currently is on the faculty at Southern California. Lewis explains, "Our main interest was to determine the reliability of the ratings. This was equal-appearing-intervals rating on a nine-point scale." So he and Grings selected ninety-six samples from the Dassler recordings, and had large numbers of students rate them to get the reliability: "That's a correlational procedure and we found fairly high reliability." Then Grings was drafted.

> I tried to get somebody in speech pathology interested in this, to put it in some sort of form. And nobody would be interested. One of the best illustrations of resistance to it came from Joe Sheehan, a graduate student here then. I tried to explain it to him and he said, "Well, this is just voice. This isn't what you see." And I said, "That's right, but that's not what we are getting at. We are trying to see whether or not we can measure severity reliably from what is heard, on the basis of these recordings. If we can then we have accomplished something." His retort was, "Well, that won't do, that won't do!" and he walked out.

And there the story is interrupted. Lewis went into the service soon and was not to go on with this particular project until 1946.

WARTIME

A prefatory note, "In the Service," in the 1941-42 catalogue sets the scene: The University, for the fourth time in its ninety-five years, was "to muster its resources to meet its wartime responsibility to the nation." From then on course listings are sprinkled with an ever increasing number of italic lines: *omitted in 1942-43* (or whatever the year)—another faculty member was in the service. There were also new wartime courses and research projects, accelerated courses, nonresident courses, special offerings to accommodate the Navy Preflight Program established here in April 1942, and, later on, others to accommodate returning veterans.

The war years were a time of stress and distress for the Program as well as for the entire University community. Fairbanks was one of the first faculty people directly connected with the Program to leave. He spent part of 1943 in war-related research for the Psychological Corporation, and was in uniform from 1944 to 1946 as chief of the army's aural rehabilitation section, Borden General Hospital, Chickasha, Oklahoma. Knott was a navy officer for two years, Lewis was a liaison officer with the signal corps, Stuit was a navy officer, and Keaster was associated with Fairbanks at Borden for the 1944-45 academic year. Strother was unsuccessful in enlisting because his work at the University was declared essential to the war effort.

Among the students in uniform were four who would become faculty members within the Program in the decade: Curtis, Frederic L. Darley, Spriestersbach, and Earl Schubert. The first three received their M.A.s in 1940. Darley and Spriestersbach went into the service then, Curtis after his Ph.D. in 1942, and Schubert after the M.S. the same year.

MEMO

It was early in 1943, when wartime stresses were beginning to develop, that Johnson wrote Mabie an unusual memo.[1] It was thirty-nine pages long, and it was a look to the future. It centered on a request for more research assistants and more research funds, even as students and faculty were leaving daily to go into uniform or to serve as specialists in war-related activities. It becomes memorable as a statement of accomplishments, problems, and philosophy. And perhaps its language would have been even stronger if it had been written a few months later, because by then Fairbanks was gone. His going obviously would have made the request for help even more urgent.

Johnson began his memo: "Iowa's leadership in the speech pathology field is, I believe, generally conceded. And it is clearly recognized that this is due mainly to the research that has been done here."

Then he continues:

> In 1938 the International Council for Exceptional Children published a survey in which it was shown that over a 10-year period more studies (M.A. and Ph.D. research) had been done on the problem of exceptional children at the University of Iowa than at any other American university. Columbia was a close second and between it and the third place institution there was a large gap.
>
> I should judge that 80 to 90 per cent of the Iowa studies had been

done in speech pathology. Actually, nearly three-fourths of them had been done on stuttering. I should estimate that 75 to 80 per cent of all studies made on stuttering since 1925 have been made here in our own laboratories. Over the past four or five years a major share of the best research on articulation has been done here by Dr. Fairbanks. The basic voice research carried out over the years by Dean Seashore and his students, and the neuropsychological studies of Dr. Travis, extended in recent years by Dr. Knott, are the other chief research contributions to speech pathology by means of which Iowa has achieved and held leadership in this field.

Research as the Key. He goes on to explain how much less time the faculty had for research than in former years, and echoes words Travis and Seashore had used so many times: the key to it all is research. "Up to 1935 or 1936," he writes,

there were many more assistants in the Clinic than we now have. In 1934-35 I was devoting most of my time to work on stuttering, and, besides myself, Van Riper, Milisen, Steer, Knott, Brown, and Bagchi, all superior students who have since distinguished themselves, were assistants in the Clinic and they were all working with stutterers. This may sound fantastic now—*but it produced research results,* it represented a policy that put Iowa-trained directors in 25 or more college and university speech clinics over the country, it gave Iowa a dominant place in the American Speech Correction Association. It got results. I should say it was a wise policy. I urge that it be revived to the greatest possible extent.

I am convinced that Strother, Fairbanks and myself are spending altogether too much time in teaching and in handling cases. There may be points of view from which this is justified or even desirable, but it will jeopardize Iowa's position of leadership in speech pathology if it is continued. We should have more assistants. Fairbanks now has none, Strother has two, I have two. There used to be seven or eight, and in the meantime our program has grown. Economy argues against adding more research assistants. The requirements of high grade instruction and research leadership argue for it. . . .

I have plans for a comprehensive program of research on stuttering. After the war I should hope to obtain funds, perhaps from outside sources, with which to make a broad and systematic attack on this problem particularly and on other problems related to it. Strother, Fairbanks, and Reger also have research plans along their particular lines of specialization. I hope that administrative policy will favor the rigorous execution of these plans, by means of a realistic adjustment of teaching schedules, and budgetary provisions for assistants and equipment.

Perhaps I have said enough, but I want to leave no doubt whatever as to my own point of view, at least. Practically any university can maintain a teacher-training and clinical service program in speech pathology. There is really no source of distinction in that, nor is there any possibility for making a major or basic contribution. The university that maintains leadership in research can well afford to let other institutions surpass it along lines of applied speech pathology, because by its creative contributions it will determine the character and the value of the work they do. I would apply the same principle to the question of policy regarding our services to the state.

We can best serve Iowa by emphasizing research, because by doing that we will be providing our students with scientific training in the best sense. After all, the choice, from a public service point of view, lies between having our major staff members give help directly to a few dozen cases a year, or enabling them to produce the scientific data and methods whereby their students can give help not to dozens but to hundreds or thousands of cases per year.

We can best discharge our responsibility to the public by turning out scientifically oriented graduates, equipped with the knowledge and techniques that only research can produce, who will then be adequately prepared to do the practical clinical work that the people of the state want done. If we try to do this practical work ourselves the scientific job will not be done, and in the end everyone will be the loser.

ANOTHER VIEW

Hildred Schuell,[2] who in 1946 was to become director of the aphasia section of the neurology service, Minneapolis Veterans Administration Hospital, and in 1950, professor of Neurology, University of Minnesota Graduate School of Medicine, arrived in Iowa City as a doctoral candidate in the summer of 1943, the year of the Johnson memo (above). Not long before her death in 1970 she was asked about her recollections of the Strother period. Her answer *(15)*, which in a way complements the memo, was this word picture of an era:

If I came to Iowa City today as I came in the summer of 1943, with an academic background in classics, arts, and humanities, I would surely not be accepted as a doctoral candidate in Speech Pathology. I came because I had encountered pupils with speech defects in public schools, and thought someone should know what to do. I'd had ten hours of course work in the Indiana University Extension Center in South Bend taught by Dr. Milisen and Dr. Van Riper, and I came with a letter of introduction from Dr. Van Riper. I registered as a Ph.D. candidate because I had an M.A., thought a Ph.D. came next in the natural course of events.

Dr. Mabie, who had not had a student who had read Greek drama in Greek or studied Shakespeare under a great Shakespearian scholar, tried to persuade me to major in play-writing, saying there was no future for a woman in Speech Pathology. Wendell Johnson, however, said he thought Speech Pathology was enriched by students with diverse academic backgrounds. As a matter of fact this background was relevant to later study of linguistics.

The exciting thing I got from Wendell Johnson was my first insight into the philosophy and methods of science. This was one of the most profound intellectual experiences I have ever had. I had not known that knowledge was tentative and subject to revision, how it accrued, or by what criteria it could be evaluated. It seemed to me I was learning how to think for the first time. I learned in Wendell's classes, from reading, and from hours of discussion in his seminars, over my dissertation, and in the casual day to day interchanges of ideas we had here and there, and which continued until his death.

There were other sources of stimulation. I learned about design of experiments and scientific writing from Dr. Spence's course in learning theory. I took anatomy of the ear and larynx from Dr. Scheldrup, and to my surprise found myself fascinated by beauty of structure and precise anatomical detail.

I took courses in psychometrics and organic disorders from Dr. Strother. I had expected these to be dull, but I was enthralled by his thorough and penetrating scholarship, and the sensitivity of his clinical observation. I was particularly stimulated by his course on aphasia, in which he carefully and critically delineated what was known and what was not known about the brain, about language, and about aphasia. He introduced us to the Medical Library, where I read Hughlings Jackson, Sherrington, and Fulton. He assigned me to give psychometric tests to all the children in ungraded rooms in Iowa City Schools, and to analyze the different kinds of profiles they presented. This experience, together with administering tests in the Out-Patient Clinic Tuesday afternoons, introduced me to much of the methodology I later used to explore aphasic disabilities.

Other valuable experiences came from attending Dr. Lierle's Friday afternoon clinics in the hospital. Every Friday he demonstrated to us and to his residents that the significant thing about hearing loss was the way it interfered with the development of a child or the human capacities of an adult, and that this was the proper concern of the otolaryngologist, the audiologist, the psychologist, and the speech pathologist. We began to get glimpses of the fact that speech and hearing processes are inseparable, although at the time I was not much interested in hearing.

Dr. Seashore was Acting Dean of the Graduate School the year I spent in Iowa City. He himself was a classical scholar, and because I had once read Greek, he often took time to talk to me when I visited the Graduate School offices. We talked of many things, but often of what speech pathology was about. He was always aware that we do not know enough, and that we had to cross disciplines to obtain the kind of knowledge we needed. He thought we needed to know more about language, more about perception, more about physiology, neurology, and behavior than was yet known. This made a deep impression on me, and I have never forgotten it.

Once Wendell Johnson said, "A Ph.D. doesn't mean very much. You just do a certain amount of work and eventually they decide you've done enough and give you a Ph.D., and you go on from there. It's a beginning, not an end."

I think that was the climate. We went out knowing we didn't know very much, as in truth we didn't, but we knew we could find out more, and that this was somehow the most exciting thing in the world. We had a negligible background in statistics and instrumentation, but we were oriented to thinking in terms of problems, taught to ask significant questions, and to consider the kinds of methods that were relevant to obtaining answers, which we regarded as partial and tentative. Grant Fairbanks was in the army while I was at Iowa. I regretted this much more later, when I had experienced the joy of his beautifully lucid thinking. I think I missed a lot by not having had his courses; on the other hand it's possible that I wasn't yet ready for experimental phonetics.

AN "OFF-CAMPUS PROGRAM"

Curtis's *(1)* wartime experiences sound almost like an off-campus Iowa Program. After his 1942 Ph.D. under Fairbanks, he served two years as a civilian specialist and two years as a navy officer. His first assignment in the former capacity was to substitute for Iowa-trained Mack Steer in the speech clinic at Purdue after Steer joined the navy. Then he joined Fairbanks on the staff of a research project on military communications in Washington. Next he was sent to Harvard to become a member of the psychoacoustics laboratory staff and speech communications research group. From there he was sent to the army air force speech communications project in Waco, Texas, to serve as laboratory director. The project director there was Iowa-trained John Black, and the signal corps liaison officer from Washington with whom they worked was Don Lewis.

After a year in the Waco laboratory, studying ways and means of improving communication under conditions of noise, he received a commission as a navy officer and was assigned to the Bureau of Naval Personnel Research unit. Head of the unit was Iowa's Dewey Stuit. (William Maucker, for many years president of the University of Northern Iowa, was also in the unit.) Curtis was assigned to evaluate personnel selection tests and performance tests in specified situations—in choosing crews for small boats and submarines, for example. (At one point he went on a sixty-eight hour test dive of a submarine called the Sailfish which was, in fact, the renowned Squalus, raised and refitted. Later he helped test captured optical equipment and, finally, worked on personnel selection and performance tests as a member of the United States Navy Advisory Group in China, whose assignment was to help China develop a modern navy.

CURRICULUM

There were regular listings of a full course of study in the catalogues through the Strother period in spite of all the complications. While in many cases the listings are not too unlike those of the Travis period, there are differences to suggest that, as Johnson had insisted, research was not being emphasized as it once had been. There is also evidence of increased emphasis on clinical work, and certainly on both classroom and clinical work with organic speech disorders. There is also the new point of view represented by general semantics as a course and as an orientation.

Strother taught Travis introductory course at first; later, *Johnson* did. The two men taught the speech pathology seminar, and then *Fairbanks* joined them until he left for the service.

Beginning in 1940 Strother taught the introduction to clinical practice in speech correction and, with Johnson, Fairbanks, Reger, and Stuit, taught advanced clinical practice. From 1941 on he taught a course in organic disorders of speech and, with Johnson and Stuit, a course in the foundations of clinical psychology. Throughout the period he, Johnson, and Stuit gave individual instruction in the clinic in personal adjustment, speech, and reading, respectively. In 1943 Maude McBroom of the College of Education assisted in clinical work in reading. Beginning in 1941 Strother, Johnson, and Fairbanks, then Lynch, gave individual instruction in the Speech Department clinic. He gave a course in personality and adjustment one year, 1941-42. From 1943 on he was in charge of a practicum in clinical psychology.

Beginning in 1939 *Johnson* taught general semantics and a course in stuttering therapy and clinical practice. And for the 1939-40 year he taught problems in the psychology of speech and language, and methods in remedial speech, both of which he had introduced in the interim year. In its initial entry in the catalogue the methods course is described as "practice under supervision in the examination, diagnosis, and remedial instruction of individuals with various types of speech disorders." The description continues, "This is a teacher-training course designed especially for students who are preparing to become public school speech correction teachers. The practice teaching is supplemented with lectures, readings, and demonstrations."

This description is a sign of the times. The Iowa Program had been training public school speech clinicians from the beginning, but most of them had gone outside to Iowa to work. Only now were they beginning to find positions in Iowa in any number because the state was developing legislation to establish a public school speech and hearing program. For years Dean Seashore, Travis, Reger, Johnson, and others had worked toward one. It finally took shape through legislative action in the early forties *(2)*, by which time twenty-five other states also "had statutes relating to the education of children with speech defects."

Strother, Johnson, and *Reger,* beginning in 1945, taught a course called Clinical Practice in Speech and Hearing Disorders. For most of the period Johnson also offered coursework at the Research Station in speech correction training for teachers. Until 1945 it was a course in speech correction for preschool teachers. At the end of the period it was the introductory course, listed also in Speech and Psychology.

Reger continued his course, begun in the Travis years, in audiometric procedures. *Knott,* who was in the navy from 1944 to 1946, gave a course in neuropsychology before and after that, and taught physiological psychology from 1939 to 1967. He moved from Psychology to a full-time appointment in Psychiatry in 1946.

Fairbanks taught voice and phonetics on both the undergraduate and the graduate levels, and gave a course in experimental phonetics beginning in the Travis years and continuing until he left the campus for war service. Beginning in 1939 he also gave coursework dealing with voice and articulation disorders. He was off campus, in uniform or doing civilian research for the armed services, from 1943 on. In 1943 *Lynch* assisted in experimental phonetics, and in 1944 in voice and articulation disorders. Beginning in 1946 *Curtis* and *Lynch* are listed for both of these courses. *Keaster* taught speech for the hard of hearing and lip reading from 1945 on. Hers was the first regular offering at the University of work in lip reading. Up to this time any instruction in that area had been given only in the summer session and only by visiting faculty.

Dr. Scheldrup taught the Speech Department's course on the anatomy of the ear and vocal organs from the beginning of the period. In 1946 he was joined by Dr. W. R. Ingram. This is the course, originally on the anatomy of the ear alone, that was for many years taught by Dr. MacEwen when the Iowa Program was beginning.

Most of these courses appeared in the Psychology or the Speech Department listings, many in both. It is to be understood, however, that catalogue listings, which are the source of the information in this curriculum section, may not give a completely adequate or accurate picture of the actual work. Courses may be listed and not given. Others may be given, but with content different from that suggested in the descriptive text. Within those limitations, however, the listings at least suggest the outline of classroom work of the period.

1946

The Program Finally "In". The catalogue for 1946 was a special one because, with wartime paper restrictions, it was made to serve two years instead of one. But it was special also in another way. It was the first University of Iowa catalogue to carry any kind of a grouping of courses within the Program and to identify them as such. The listing is incomplete, because it includes only a part of those in Psychology and none of those in Speech or other departments. But it is a beginning. The identifying title is "Speech Pathology and Hearing Conservation."

In the grouping are Johnson's course in general semantics, speech pathology I and II, stuttering therapy and clinical practice, Strother's organic disorders of speech, the Strother-Johnson seminar in speech pathology, Reger's course in audiometry and hearing aids, and the practicum in speech and hearing disorders, listed for Johnson, Strother, and Reger.

Beginning and End. There is a notable coincidence here. This first catalogue listing of an enterprise so shaped by the genius of Seashore is dated 1946. And it was in 1946 that Seashore, after four years of wartime duty as acting dean of the Graduate College, retired for the second time.

A Faculty of Three Plus Two. When the war was over Fairbanks decided to accept an offer from the University of Southern California rather than return to Iowa. His relations with Mabie had been strained, and he was not pleased with Mabie's postwar plans for speech science. He taught at USC for two years, then moved to the University of Illinois, and later went to the Stanford Research Institute, where he was serving at the time of his death in 1964.

Fairbanks's decision not to return to Iowa meant, among other things, that Curtis, now out of uniform, had an offer of faculty appointment from Iowa, as well as from Princeton and the University of Pittsburgh. He found the choice difficult to make but finally, concluding that "personal ties and the part of yourself that you leave in graduate college are pretty important," he decided on Iowa. He returned here in 1946 as an associate professor in the Department of Speech.

And so it was that the faculty for the Program in 1946 was three full-time people, Strother, Johnson, and Curtis, plus Reger and Keaster. Reger, though full-time on the Otolaryngology budget, was shared with the Program. Keaster, full-time in a joint appointment in Otolaryngology and Speech, divided her days between the Program and Otolaryngology.

Speech Science. Curtis's position on the faculty was as successor to Grant Fairbanks, and therefore in speech science, which he proceeded to develop as a major area in the Program and in the Department of Speech. In the beginning he was, in effect, building on the foundation of work Fairbanks had done before he went into the service.

Lynch, who had taught with Fairbanks, and who had continued in speech science through the war, was now able to shift back to general speech, where her particular interest was speech excellence in public speaking and the dramatic arts.

Residential Clinic. The summer of 1946 was the first summer of the Residential Clinic. Or, perhaps a better way to say that is to say that 1946 was the year in which the summer clinic became a residential clinic. There had been summer speech work for children almost from the beginning of the Program because word of the Iowa work got around and parents began to bring or send their children to Iowa City during summer vacation to get help with speech problems. Arrangements for housing and other needs were made by the parents on an individual basis.

Strother remembers that there were children around during the summers he was here as a student. Darley remembers *(2)* them as early as 1940; so does Mrs. Earl Schubert *(14).* Jeanne Smith says *(17)* that as early as 1938 selected children from the Annie Wittenmeyer Home in Davenport were here, too, staying in foster homes like the rest.

In 1946, however, a combination of circumstances led to the beginning of a residential program. The Earl Schuberts had been married that spring, when he was discharged from the service, and wanted to return to the campus to finish graduate work. But no housing was available. In that day, with veterans returning to the campus, the demand for housing was so great that all the University units were reserved for graduate students with one or more children, and for faculty members being hired to handle the burgeoning post-war enrollment.

Mrs. Schubert tells how she and her husband finally got a roof over their heads: "When Professor Don Lewis suggested we contact Professor Gladys Lynch about the possibility of acquiring an 'instant' family and housing at the same time, it seemed a logical solution to both the needs of the residence program and our desire to return to graduate school."

And so it was that the Schuberts had a place to live and had a "family" of about two dozen boys, aged five through sixteen, living in Howard House, and about the same number of girls of about the same ages next door in McChesney House. These houses, at 8 and 12 East Bloomington, were University properties.

Mrs. Schubert remembers that first summer at Howard House as "a great experience, to say the least, and in many ways rewarding beyond any venture undertaken before or since. Because of the needs which surfaced that first summer, including an outbreak of the mumps, the following year brought forth additions and modifications to the program so that our subsequent summers as parents seemed somewhat like child's play."

The summer of 1946, then, was the first for the Residential Summer

Clinic, it was the year that Curtis joined the faculty to succeed Fairbanks, and in a few months it also became the year of the coal strike, remembered by many because of the chilly classrooms.

Scaling Again. It was in 1946 that Lewis returned to the campus after his war service. Dorothy Sherman was then in Iowa City, called here by the death of her father. She enrolled for graduate work, began taking courses in psychology, among them Lewis's logic of measurement and scaling, and became interested in the scaling problem, for which Lewis had found so little enthusiasm from others before the war. "She has gone on from there. She has done many, many very fine studies."

Recalling those earlier experiences in this research, Lewis adds, "I am not saying that the frequency of occurrence of stuttering is not a useful measure. It is, in certain ways. But I think that we found, especially Trotter found [William Trotter, M.A. 1950, Ph.D. 1953], that the measurement of severity, even though for a very short interval, was useful in seeing some of the trend lines for severity over successive readings and that sort of thing. Well, that was the beginning." And again the story rests for awhile.

New Counseling Service. Strother and Johnson had been using most of their uncommitted time for many years to counsel students with adjustment problems, as Johnson wrote some years later *(5).* With the help of others who were interested, and after their own extended effort over a long period of time, they finally saw the University establish the Student Counseling office in 1946. The Counseling Office was staffed with "clinical psychologists who assumed official responsibility for the psychological counseling of students with personal problems." These psychologists, it will be remembered, would have been trained at least partially in coursework and procedures to which Strother had contributed in his larger engagement with the new discipline.

STUTTERING AND GENERAL SEMANTICS

Johnson's research and clinical work in stuttering, his prolific writing, and his work in general semantics were all going forward simultaneously, each affecting the others. He was involved particularly in studies of the onset of stuttering *(9),* and with research and clinical procedures in which the role of language ("We create our world linguistically, how else?") and speaker-listener interactions *(20,* pp. 897-915) were seen as fundamental factors ("A stutterer has four legs"). These studies were concerned not only with stuttering but also with other speech problems and, more broadly, with language and the process of communication. ("The speaker is often his most enchanted listener.")

During this period Johnson wrote *People in Quandaries (7)* as a text for his class in general semantics. It was more than that. It was a statement of his position on the use of the principles of general semantics in dealing with problems in human behavior, including stuttering. From this time on he emphasized the centrality of communication in human relations, often using his research and clinical experience in stuttering as a point of departure.

In 1943 he was among those responsible for the establishment of *ETC., a Review of General Semantics,* by the International Society for General Semantics. (He served on its editorial board from the founding until 1958.) He published in that quarterly many times, beginning with the very first issue (August 1943) which included his "You Can't Write Writing," an article reprinted many times down through the years (e.g., S. I. Hayakawa, Ed., *Language, Meaning, and Maturity, Selections from ETC., a Review of General Semantics, 1943-1953,* New York: Harper & Row, 1954).

Through 1938 he had published thirty-five articles and the book, *Because I Stutter (6).* From 1939 through 1947 he published thirty articles as well as *People in Quandaries,* most of them related to stuttering. His bibliography of University of Iowa studies of stuttering (*8*, pp. 447-63) shows thirty-nine publications by his students during the period.

AUDIOLOGY

The Strother period was the period in which "audiology" appeared on the scene as a word and as a new discipline in an area close to the Iowa Program and, nationally, in areas related to both speech pathology and clinical psychology.

The word *(13)* was apparently introduced by Dr. Ray Carhart and Dr. Norton Canfield as the name for this new science which was growing out of war-related aural rehabilitation projects, and which for years had been developing at Iowa in Otolaryngology. The science was supported by a growing literature which included, as if to bind the past with the present, a book by C. C. Bunch, Seashore's first "psychologist of otology," who devoted his professional life to an effort to gain recognition for clinical audiology as a science. He died in 1941. His book, called *Clinical Audiology,* was published posthumously, by Mosby, St. Louis, in 1943. (A tribute to Bunch and his work was written by Clarence Simon, another early day Iowan, for the March 1943 issue of the *Journal of Speech Disorders.*)

Indications of the growing interest in this new science at Iowa in the Strother period were the classroom and laboratory activity during the regular school year and the joint sponsorship, by Otolaryngology, Speech, and Psychology, of graduate-level coursework at summer session workshops in hearing conservation. In a 1944 memo Johnson describes that summer's workshop as a "training course in audiology and the fitting of hearing aids," with "weekly lectures and discussions on speech and hearing rehabilitation by outstanding authorities." This workshop lasted four weeks. Guest lecturers were Bryng Bryngelson of Minnesota, Herbert Koepp-Baker and Harold Westlake of Penn State, and Raymond Carhart of Northwestern. Dr. Lierle and Reger of the Iowa faculty took a particularly active part.

These two men carried leadership roles in the new field nationally as well as locally, beginning in the early forties when Dr. Lierle was chairman of the committee on the conservation of hearing of the American Academy of Ophthalmology and Otolaryngology. (His final report as chairman of the committee was written in October 1968,[3] an impressive document in which twelve major national enterprises are listed among committee projects.) One of the first projects that the committee devoted itself to was the testing of hearing of school children. Reger and Dr. Horace Newhart of Minneapolis produced a manual of conservation-of-hearing procedures for public school systems which, in its time, was said to be the one and only standardization of hearing test procedures and of criteria of hearing impairment in relation to severity. It was published *(12)* as a supplement to the transactions of the Academy in 1945, then revised and published a second time in 1956.

To prepare the original draft Reger went up to Dr. Newhart's home two or three times to work with him there, and Dr. Newhart came down here two or three times to work with Reger. Then the two presented their proposed draft to Dr. Lierle's committee, heads of departments and research people in hearing who represented most parts of the United States. "We read it to them chapter by chapter," Reger recalls,

and this was almost drudgery. And these specialists discussed it and criticized it, and questioned us, point by point.

The two of us really put our opinions and reputations on the line in this manual, for instance when we said that we felt that a hearing loss of 15 dB could be a significant loss. Now today I think that's 10 dB. But you see, more is known about testing. We have better earphone cushions today that exclude noise, and now we have noise-level meters to measure what the noise environment is, and so on. We had none of that then. We knew that if a person had a flat 30 dB loss in both ears, this person was beginning to have trouble in understanding speech. We had observed this.

Meanwhile, the war itself was not only making audiology a science but was bringing speech pathology and audiology together. Iowa's Newby, for years professor and director of speech pathology and audiology in Stanford University's School of Medicine, and later at the University of Maryland, wrote of this in his book called *Audiology* (*13,* pp. 1-2). He called audiology

the offspring of two parents: speech pathology and otology. Speech pathology deals with the diagnosis and treatment of individuals who suffer from disorders in oral language. Otology is concerned with the diagnosis and treatment of individuals who have an ear disease or disorders of the peripheral mechanism of hearing. Speech pathology is primarily a nonmedical specialty, whereas otology is purely a medical specialty. . . . The two fields of speech pathology and otology were wedded in World War II in the so-called aural rehabilitation centers established by the armed forces for the benefit of hearing-impaired personnel.

The care and rehabilitation of these people required the closest team-work between medical and nonmedical specialists. Some nonmedical persons recruited for work in aural rehabilitation centers were teachers of the deaf, but for the most part they were people whose training and experience had been in the field of speech pathology and speech correction. Now in the aural rehabilitation centers, they extended their responsibilities to the development of tests of hearing function, selection of hearing aids, and the development of various rehabilitative techniques which extended far beyond speech correction.

Thus through the cooperative efforts of the two specialties of speech pathology and otology, a new field of specialization was created. Although there had been notable examples of individuals who devoted themselves to working with the hard of hearing before the 1940's the professional field of audiology did not exist until World War II.

It is of interest to note here that in 1947 the American Speech Correction Association became the American Speech and Hearing Association, and its *Journal of Speech Disorders* became the *Journal of Speech and Hearing Disorders*.

STROTHER AND THE HOSPITAL SCHOOL

The University's Hospital School is a direct descendant of projects in which Strother was involved early in the war. When he assumed responsibility for the psychological clinic in the Psychopathic Hospital, and for clinical services at the General Hospital and the Children's Hospital, there was, he explains,

a convalescent home for crippled children that was run by the department of orthopedics in Children's Hospital as a part of the Crippled Children's Services. Dr. Steindler was actively involved in this. I had the clinic over in East Hall and also I had the clinic in Psychopathic Hospital and worked with the Children's Hospital and the General Hospital, particularly Dr. Lierle's department in General Hospital, and pediatrics and orthopedics in Children's Hospital. My work was in both clinical psychology and speech pathology.

Dr. Theodore J. Gretteman of orthopedics, Dr. Robert Jackson of Pediatrics, and Strother were all associated with the Iowa Society for Crippled Children at the time. The secretary was Dorothy Phillips. The four attended a meeting in Chicago of the National Society for Crippled Children and Adults. Strother remembers that on the way back on the train they got to talking about the need for a hospital school. This would have been in 1945 or 1946: "So we got quite interested in this possibility. The four of us then drafted the initial legislation for the hospital school," Strother recalls.

> And then when it approached time for the legislature, we had to consider attempting to get official University approval for this and work out the legislative campaign for it.
>
> I approached President Hancher and asked if he would endorse this. And he was quite reluctant to do so because he felt that if this appropriation were connected with the University it might detract from other capital needs that the University had, and also that the cost of operation would be charged against the University budget.
>
> So it was decided that it would be better to set this up as something quite separate from the University, and request a distinct appropriation for a State Hospital School located at the University and affiliated with it, but not controlled by it. With this agreement, then, we went into the legislature, and Dorothy Phillips, I think, deserves the primary credit for the lobbying. She managed the campaign in the legislature.
>
> Finally the legislature approved the school and even offered more money than we were asking since by then a quite favorable climate of opinion had built up. So the initial appropriation was made, and this was the beginning of the Hospital School.

The legislative enactment was in 1947, about a year after the conversation on the train coming back from Chicago. (The school took its first child in October 1948, in temporary quarters in Westlawn. The first admissions in the new building were in January 1954. Dr. R. R. Rembolt was medical director in 1948, became director of the school in 1952, and has continued in that position.)

AN HISTORIC CONFERENCE

Strother, as a representative of the University of Iowa, participated in the historic Boulder Conference of 1947, at which the pattern was set for subsequent graduate programs in clinical psychology. The conference was called by the United States Public Health Service, the Veterans Administration, and the American Psychological Association to develop guidelines for such programs. Proceedings were published by the APA under the editorship of Victor Raimy (*Conference on Graduate Education in Clinical Psychology,* New York: Prentice-Hall, 1950).

MORE ON THE NATIONAL LEVEL

Other activities on the national level in this period included presidential administrations of four former Iowans in the affairs of the American Speech Correction Association and its successor, the American Speech and Hearing Association. Sara Hawk was president in 1939 and 1940, Bryngelson the following two years, Simon in 1946, and Koepp-Baker in 1947.

Johnson became president of the International Society for General Semantics in 1945, and served a four-year term. He was also editor of the *Journal of Speech Disorders* from 1943 on, through the Strother period.

And in this second period of the Iowa Program, three of its leaders received the Honors of the Association of the American Speech and Hearing Association: Seashore in 1944, the first time the award was given; Johnson in 1946; and Travis in 1947.

STROTHER RESIGNS

The war had been over for about a year when the University of Washington asked Strother to return. Perhaps the timing had something to do with his decision or perhaps, as he suspects now, his heart had always been back there and he had missed the mountains and the ocean. In any case, he found himself so drawn by the opportunity to develop an entire new program in clinical psychology that he accepted Washington's invitation and went back to Seattle in the summer of 1947. Strother has remained on the Washington faculty, holding a joint appointment in the Department of Psychology and the Department of Psychiatry. His principal work is as director of the University's renowned Mental Retardation and Child Development Center, built by Strother and his colleagues.

REFERENCES

1. James F. Curtis, taped conversations with author, June and November 1968, January 1969, January 1972.

2. Frederic L. Darley, personal correspondence with author, January 30, 1969.

3. Dorothy Ann Eckelmann, "A Handbook of Public School Speech Correction," Ph.D. dissertation, University of Iowa, 1952.

4. Editors, "In Memoriam, Wendell Johnson, 1906-1965," *General Semantics Bulletin, 32* and *33,* 1965/1966, 133-146.

5. Wendell Johnson, "Are Speech Disorders 'Superficial' or 'Basic'?" *Asha, 3,* August 1961, 233-236.

6. Wendell Johnson, *Because I Stutter* (New York: Appleton, 1930).

7. Wendell Johnson, *People in Quandaries,* (New York: Harper & Row, 1946).

8. Wendell Johnson (Ed.), *Stuttering in Children and Adults* (Minneapolis: University of Minnesota Press, 1955).

9. Wendell Johnson and Associates, *The Onset of Stuttering* (Minneapolis: University of Minnesota Press, 1959).

10. Wendell Johnson, James Curtis, Spencer Brown, Jacqueline Keaster, and Clarence Edney, *Speech Handicapped School Children* (New York: Harper & Row, 1948, 1956, 1967): Johnson (Ed.), 1948, 1956; Johnson and Dorothy Moeller (Eds.), 1967.

11. Don Lewis, taped conversation with author, Iowa City, October 1, 1969.

12. Horace Newhart and Scott Reger, *Manual for a School Hearing Conservation Program* (Rochester, Minnesota: American Academy of Ophthalmology and Otolaryngology [supplement to Academy's Transactions], 1945, revised 1956).

13. Hayes Newby, *Audiology: Principles and Practice* (New York: Appleton-Century-Crofts, 1958).

14. Mrs. Earl Schubert, personal correspondence with author, May 24, 1969.

15. Hildred Schuell, *Differences Which Matter: a Study of Boys and Girls* (Austin, Texas: Delta Kappa Gamma Society, 1947).

16. Hildred Schuell, personal correspondence with author, March 25, 1968.

17. Jeanne Kellenberger Smith, conversations and personal correspondence with author, October and November 1971, March 1972.

18. Bette Rae Bartell Spriestersbach, conversation with author, November 1968.

19. Charles Strother, taped conversation with author, Chicago, March 1, 1968, and personal correspondence with author, February 16, 1971, April 1972, and subsequent correspondence.

20. Lee Edward Travis (Ed.), *Handbook of Speech Pathology* (New York: Appleton-Century-Crofts, 1957).

NOTES

[1] Memos in this chapter, unless otherwise identified, are from official records filed in University archives in the University Library.

[2] She was the originator of the well-known phrase, "the clinical point of view in education," which she had used in her own writing *(15),* and which has been used

widely by others—including Johnson, who makes it a chapter title in *Speech Handicapped School Children (10)*.

[3] A copy of this report is filed in the archives of the Department of Speech Pathology and Audiology. It is also available in Dr. Lierle's office and in official documents of the Academy.

7

THE JOHNSON PERIOD: 1947-1955

The third period in the history of the Iowa Program in Speech Pathology and Audiology began in the fall of 1947, when Wendell Johnson succeeded Charles Strother as principal officer. It continued until the spring of 1955 when Johnson, regaining strength after a heart attack the previous December, chose to relinquish his administrative duties. For a decade longer, however, he was able to continue as an active member of the faculty in what he liked to call his creative venturing—teaching, counseling, lecturing, writing, and consulting. He died in 1965.

A person of unusual sensitivity to human needs, who by then had fought his own way from relative speechlessness to relative fluency, Johnson was already well and widely known when he assumed his new office. He was then in his fifth year as editor of the *Journal of Speech Disorders* of the American Speech and Hearing Association, was on the Association's executive council, had received the Association's Honors award the year before, had been a founder of the ASHA Speech Correction Fund the year before that, was completing his term as president of the International Society for General Semantics, was on the Society's editorial and governing boards, was on the board of the Institute of General Semantics as well, had authored or co-authored sixty-two articles, and had written two books, *Because I Stutter,* and *People in Quandaries.*

During his administration Iowa came to be called the stuttering capital of the world, and perhaps it was. But that term, "stuttering capital," omits much, for the Program developed broadly and in important ways to include speech science, audiology, speech disorders other than stuttering, and pioneering psychosocial research in human speech problems. In this period the Program at last acquired a measure of autonomy instead of being a "free-floating entity," as James Curtis *(1)* on occasion described it.

Once again, as in the administrations of Travis and Strother, there was evident a harmony between the interests of the chief officer and the content of the Program. Travis had been the innovator in the great pioneering research thrust that demonstrated that speech behavior could be quantified as well as qualified. Strother had given new emphasis to work with organic speech disorders, a change that strengthened the Program through new kinds of contacts with health-related sciences and agencies both within and beyond the University community, thus broadening the already robust interdisciplinary element of the Program. Johnson invested himself in a notable and vigorous effort to understand the problem of stuttering. As time went on he sought this understanding less within the limits of a specific speech disorder, and more in terms of *(4)* "the relation of our ways of talking to our ways of life." His interpretation of the general semantics approach to the effective handling of human problems—that is, the teaming of the creative and directive force of language with the method of science—was reflected in the many facets of his work. With his encouragement Iowa's great body of stuttering research and publication grew *(7,* pp. 447-463), with much of the work in this period being concerned also with the relation of human speaking behavior to other human behaviors. A sense of search undergirded all of this. As he put it in his notes for a talk at the 1950 ASHA convention, "The biggest change in my orientation to the stuttering problem in the past 20 years is that 20 years ago I thought I knew all the answers and today I am beginning to suspect that I might know a few of the questions."

Iowa's leadership continued on the state scene, particularly in the activities of the Iowa Speech and Hearing Association and in the Iowa Society for Crippled Children and Adults. Projects with state programs, agencies, and institutions flourished.

Nationally, the faculty contributed in diverse ways to the building of speech pathology and audiology as a discipline. Such contributions were evident particularly in efforts to upgrade standards of the profession and to cultivate a public awareness of the importance of speech and language in everyday living.

One such effort was in process at the very beginning of the period, as Johnson was to note *(6)* in the March 1948 issue of the *Journal of Speech and Hearing Disorders:*

> The Speech Correction Foundation was established by action of the Council of the American Speech Correction Association December 30, 1946. It is an expression of the growing realization that there is a tremendous need for more speech correction workers, expanded clinical facilities, and intensified research.
>
> As a matter of historical interest, the Foundation, as such, grew out of efforts made by speech defectives themselves to stimulate the greater development of speech correction in the United States. In 1939 a group of stutterers at the University of Iowa organized the Demosthenes Club (named after the Greek, Demosthenes, who is credited by legend with having overcome a speech defect to become one of the greatest orators of all time).
>
> The idea spread, and soon there were chapters of the Demosthenes Club in several American cities and universities, and a chapter was formed also at the University of Witwatersrand, Johannesburg, South

Africa. As a result, the proposal was put forth that a national, or even international, organization be developed. The Iowa Chapter members prepared a preliminary draft of a constitution for such an organization which they proposed to call "The Stuttering Research Foundation," and this was presented to the Council of the American Speech Correction Association at its annual meeting in December 1945.

After that 1945 presentation the Council named a committee, with Johnson as chairman, to revise and broaden the base of the original document. It was action on the revised statement that established the Foundation. Then in 1947 and 1948 preliminary work was done, so that in 1949 the final stages of organization were completed. At that point the National Society for Crippled Children and Adults was also a sponsor. Johnson continued his interests in the project which would move into a new period of development after his Iowa administration was over.

He apparently felt very strongly about the Foundation and about the idea behind it. Two notes he wrote in December 1947 are witness to this.[1] To President Virgil M. Hancher[2] he expressed "deep satisfaction at the establishment of the Speech Correction Foundation which had its origin on this campus. . . . The first letters to activate the program are in the mail today." And to Dean Seashore he had this to say: "Your vision and inspiring leadership have yielded an abundance of fine fruits, and I now have the deep satisfaction of contributing one more bright golden orange to the harvest . . . on behalf of children and adults to be benefited I want simply and with deep feeling to thank you for making inevitable, through your wise humanitarianism and constant encouragement, the creation of this Foundation."

Postwar Challenges. The Johnson administration was characterized by notable changes in the Program's context and structure, many of these dictated, or at least given impetus, by the challenges, stresses, and strains of the postwar situation. In the first place, veterans were returning, producing a student body older and more mature than that of preceding years. In the second place, enrollment in the Program, as in the University as a whole, was increasing rapidly. Beyond all this, activities in war-associated speech and hearing rehabilitation had added to the basics in the field the entirely new science of audiology, and had introduced an array of new professional opportunities in teaching, research, and service for which graduates must now be trained. The demand on curriculum planning is obvious.

Quite understandably, it was in these years that in certain matters of day-to-day operations the advantages of interdisciplinary cooperation began to be outweighed by the disadvantages. The Program still operated under the rules and regulations and budgets of the several departments in which it had been nourished and in which, as a separate entity, it had grown. This arrangement was notably inefficient, and in the face of the new demands, it became quite unworkable. A new administrative structure was needed, and for several years Johnson gave much of his energy to establishing one.

He was faced with a subtle problem. The Program was not pulling away from its friends, it was simply seeking recognition of its own identity in the form of a reasonably efficient framework for its activities. Johnson expressed his thinking on these matters when some years later he was asked about the "general movement away from the 'speech arts' between 1925 and 1950." He had this to say *(3):*

> To the best of my knowledge it is largely a misconception that there was any movement of speech pathology and audiology as a profession away from the speech arts. At the University of Iowa where I grew up professionally the program in speech pathology and audiology was primarily the creation, originally, of Dean Carl E. Seashore, who was Dean of the Graduate College and Head of the Department of Psychology.
>
> He developed it as an interdepartmental intercollege program and from its inception in the early twenties to the establishment of the Department of Speech Pathology and Audiology in 1956, the program was not in any one department. It was sponsored primarily by the Departments of Psychology, Child Welfare, Otolaryngology, and Speech, and drew its courses from more than a dozen different departments and from the Colleges of Liberal Arts, Education, and Medicine primarily. The program was never a part of the Department of Speech and Dramatic Arts in any official sense.
>
> As I analyze the major activities, interests, and problems of speech pathologists and audiologists, on the one hand, and on the other hand, members of the field of speech and the dramatic arts, there is very little overlap. Indeed, it has been my experience that those students who have elected to transfer from a major in the speech arts to a major in speech pathology and audiology have had to undergo a very considerable readjustment, because they came from a field in which the emphasis was upon excellence in performance to a field in which the major preoccupation is with disorder and the lack of excellence, and in many cases the impossibility of achieving excellence.
>
> In my judgment, the facts are that speech pathology and audiology is a new profession and by no means an outgrowth of the speech arts or of any other older profession or academic area. It is a profession and a field of scholarship and research which has grown up in response to one of the most important of all human needs, the need to understand and minister to persons who are handicapped in respect to the only distinctively human bodily function, namely that which underlies the processes of human speech and comprehension of

speech and of communicative behavior generally.

The problems of human communication cannot be solved within the confines of any one academic department, even a department of speech pathology and audiology. Our profession draws necessarily upon all the resources and facilities of the physical, biological, behavioral, and social sciences, so far as these are relevant to the needs of the scholar and the professional worker who has the responsibility of understanding as best he can the disorders of communication that beset human beings and the factors that are related to these disorders.

THE DIVISION OF THE CLINIC

From the very beginning of the third period Johnson had one great advantage in his labors for official recognition of the autonomy of the Program. That was the formal separation of the Psychological and Speech Clinic into the Psychological Clinic and the Speech Clinic. The former became the responsibility of the Psychology Department, the latter, the responsibility of the Program.

The creation of the University counseling service may have been a factor in the decision to separate the Clinic, since certain phases of the work would logically go to the new service unit. Or the decision may have been recognition of the *de facto* separation that had existed for some time as a result of the division of the clinical caseload during Strother's administration.

Strother *(20)* feels that official separation of the Clinic brought new definition and focus to the Program. And this, in turn, he suggests, became a force for unity which helped to restore to the Program some of the cohesion it had known before the war years.

A more or less routine letter, written by President Hancher in answer to a query from a physician in Canada in October 1947, becomes a historical document in that it commits to paper, officially, the new clinic names. The president calls the Clinic the Speech Clinic, he refers to Johnson as Director of the Speech Clinic, and he describes the clinic as, "an official administrative unit of the University, sponsored by the departments of speech, psychology, and child welfare, with the cooperation of the colleges of medicine, education, and other divisions of the University."

By way of orientation to this period it is perhaps useful to remember that Strother's resignation in 1947 left Johnson and Curtis as the only full-time faculty members within the Program. Dr. Lierle continued to loan Reger even though his position was completely on the budget of the Department of Otolaryngology and Maxillofacial Surgery (until 1952 Otolaryngology and Oral Surgery, and earlier, Otology). Gladys Lynch, who had joined the Speech Department faculty in 1943, and had taught speech science with Fairbanks, now worked with Curtis in speech science, although her interests and responsibilities were more in the direction of excellence rather than pathologies of speech. Jacqueline Keaster, who had joined the faculty in 1945 after two summers as a visiting professor, held a joint appointment, dividing her time between the Program and Dr. Lierle's department.

Lewis, though supported completely by Psychology, taught a required course in the fundamentals of hearing. And Knott, since 1946 full-time in Psychiatry, had contact with the Program through his work in the area of electrophysiology and in directing graduate programs, the latter including Dean E. Williams' doctorate in 1952. This study is mentioned not only because Williams was later to join the faculty, but also because his research repeated history by being done in the Knott laboratory in the Psychopathic Hospital where Travis had had his laboratory at the very beginning of the Program, and by being concerned, as many Travis studies had been, with action potentials and stuttering. Williams worked with jaw musculature and interpreted his findings as supporting the avoidance theory rather than the so-called Orton-Travis dominance theory once favored by Travis. (Travis had by then moved away from his dominance theory and toward a theory that included psychological as well as physiological considerations.)

NEW FACULTY

New faculty members within the Johnson period were, in the order of their coming, Spencer Brown, D.C. Spriestersbach, Frederic L. Darley, Earl Schubert, Dorothy Sherman, and Charles Parker. Brown (Iowa Ph.D., 1937, Minnesota M.D., 1945) came in 1947 as associate professor in the Department of Speech, with teaching duties in the Program and major responsibility for the outpatient services of the Clinic. The Army Medical Corps had given him an early release on petition of University President Hancher, who had pointed out that Johnson was carrying on the work of the Clinic with practically no help. Brown, who had completed his medical internship at Johns Hopkins before going into the service, came back to Iowa with the understanding that he would have a joint appointment in the Program and in the College of Medicine. When this did not materialize he resigned in 1949, returning to the University of Minnesota to begin a residency in pediatrics, which he completed in 1950. Dorothy Drakesmith (Craven), later on the faculty of the University of Hawaii, held an appointment as instructor in the Program from 1949 to '51. She received her M.A. degree at Iowa in 1948.

Spriestersbach and Darley, like Brown, had returned from the service. Both had entered the program as doctoral candidates and had been assigned assistantships in the speech fundamentals course, now known as the communication skills program. Each received his faculty appointment at the time of his Ph.D., Spriestersbach in 1948, Darley in 1950.

Schubert had gone into the service as an Iowa graduate student, was on John Black's army project at Waco, and a member of Lewis's communications survey team, mostly in radar, in the South Pacific. He had come back to Iowa, completing work for his Ph.D. degree of 1948 under Lewis, and had then gone to the University of Michigan to teach. He joined the Iowa faculty in 1951 as an associate professor. Sherman came onto the faculty the same year, after completing her work for the doctorate. Parker joined the faculty after his Ph.D. in 1953. All of these new appointments were in the Speech Department. Keaster resigned to join the staff of Childrens Hospital, Los Angeles, in 1953. Her position was filled that same year by Jeanne Kellenberger Smith (Iowa M.A., 1937) whose appointment was full-time in Otolaryngology and Maxillofacial Surgery. She has worked there since that time in rehabilitative audiology, and continued in her connection with the Program as a member of its affiliated staff. Speaking recently of the growth of activities in her area as these related to speech pathology, she noted that in 1952, "the number of patients examined in Speech Pathology in Oto was 246. This number increased to 1026 in the next four years and has continued to increase, necessitating additional staff."

Johnson was continuing his teaching of general semantics, his writing, his lecturing, and his research, classroom, and clinical work—mainly with stuttering—while also serving as principal administrative officer of the Program. Curtis was in experimental phonetics, carrying forward the line which had been begun by Glenn Merry and Giles Gray, and which had then gone on through the work of Milton Metfessel, Joseph Tiffin, Fairbanks, and Lynch. He was also involved in coursework in voice and articulation disorders.

Darley succeeded to Brown's duties in both the outpatient clinic and in the area of organic speech disorders, the latter in part a continuation of Strother's work. Among other duties, Darley taught a course called introduction to clinical practice in speech correction, which was twice renamed between 1950 and 1955, first to introduction to clinical practice in speech pathology and audiology, and then to diagnosis and appraisal in speech pathology and audiology. These name changes reflected certain other changes in the developmental pattern of the Program in this period.

As director of the outpatient Clinic Darley was chairman of the social service unit in East Hall, which was administered jointly by the University and the State Department of Social Welfare. He was director of the summer residential Clinic as Brown had been before him, and he supervised the speech correction workers in the Hospital School and with the State Services for Crippled Children. Darley's teaching was in clinical procedures, diagnosis and appraisal, and organic disorders of speech. He became particularly interested in speech development and aphasia.

Spriestersbach taught the Travis-Strother-Johnson introductory course as well as courses in voice and articulation disorders, which in earlier years and other forms had been taught by Sarah Barrows, Alice Mills, Bessie Rasmus (Petersen), and Fairbanks. Soon he began teaching in the area of organic speech disorders as well, the area in which Strother had pioneered at Iowa, and it was here that his longtime interest in cleft problems began. In those early years he also had responsibility for the speech correction aspects of the communication skills program, which meant that he was supervising clinical services and a clinical staff. A memo in the early fifties indicates that this involved work for 175 University students. The staff, in addition to Spriestersbach, was one full-time instructor, two half-time instructors, a graduate assistant, and from twenty-five to forty student clinicians.

Schubert began to develop coursework in the new area of audiology. With his coming Reger could be relieved of at least a portion of the responsibility he had carried in the Program for so long, and could give more time to his primary work in Otolaryngology and Maxillofacial Surgery, where the new demands of postwar rehabilitation in hearing were adding considerably to the duties of his position. He continued to teach and to work with students in the Program, and he and Dr. Lierle cooperated generously with the Program in many ways and for many years, Reger to the present day, Dr. Lierle until 1963, when he retired. Dr. Lierle's successor, Dr. Brian McCabe, continued the tradition of cooperation.

Sherman taught courses in voice and articulation disorders, and in both methodology and practice in public school speech correction. She also worked on psychological scaling of the severity of speech disorders, continuing in the area in which she had pioneered with Lewis during her doctoral program. She became extensively involved in stuttering research as a colleague of Johnson. Parker joined Schubert in developing the curriculum in audiology.

END OF A BEGINNING

Early in the Program's sequence of comings and goings—soon after Spriestersbach had joined the faculty and only a few months after Brown left for his residency—the death of Dean Carl E. Seashore in the fall of 1949 brought to a close a great and creative career that had meant so much to the Program. "The Dean," as he was referred to with awe and affection, had carried the role of paterfamilias for three eventful, trying, and rewarding decades.

Fairbanks, then in his first year as editor of the *Journal of Speech and Hearing Disorders,* succeeding Johnson, chose to use a black-bordered picture of the Dean in the December issue (vol. 14, No. 4, p. 395) of his publication, and with it only the Seashore name, the birth and death dates: January 28, 1866, October 16, 1949. He no doubt felt that for readers of the *Journal* that was adequate. They knew Seashore. They knew his work.

In a memorial tribute in the *Psychological Review*, Tiffin *(22)*, himself a pioneer in the Program, writes of Seashore's "profound and extensive" influence on psychology and graduate study in America. He recalls also the delightful poise of this man who "went contentedly back to his laboratory when the University of Iowa chapter of Sigma Xi refused to elect him to membership during his early days at Iowa because psychology was not considered to be a science . . . (and who) took in stride his admission to the National Academy of Sciences as a representative of psychology in the early part of the century. He was the first person at the University of Iowa in any field to be so honored."

Metfessel *(14)*, also a pioneer in the program, writing of Seashore in *Science*, refers to him as a member of "that forthright and challenging group of department heads and university administrators who were pioneers in American psychology," a man "whose professional life theme . . . was a wholehearted devotion to scientific methodology in both theory and practice.

"The infusion of psychological research into the life stream of human events," Metfessel continues,

> was Dean Seashore's ideal, even at the risk that the research might ultimately lose its identity with psychology. . . . He recognized an operational meaning of the unity of the sciences, and that was in part the ground for his projects that led to the breaking down of departmental barriers. In his training programs for graduate students he made provisions for courses by specialists in other sciences: acoustics, anatomy, neurology, etc.
>
> . . . he believed that scientific theories, however verbalized and whatever the problems dealt with, should be harmonious. It happened that some of the questions asked by psychologists had not been considered by other scientists, but some kind of a reply in their terms was basic.
>
> One instance that reflected Dean Seashore's point of view was the stuttering project in the psychological clinic, under the direction of Lee Travis. The cerebral dominance theory of stuttering, although it was in the field of neurology, called for testing before the less rigidly formulated emotional theories; but it turned out to be highly restricted, and the field was left open for the latter theories. To Dean Seashore, this was just another example of the way in which science progresses by elimination of originally plausible hypotheses.
>
> . . . Some of us were fortunate to be close enough to him to share a few of his hardships and blessings. Our appreciation of the man and

his works increased steadily through the years. He helped others more than others helped him.

Dr. Lierle *(12),* long a professional colleague and close friend of the Dean, and one of his regular golfing partners, refers to Seashore as "one of the outstanding scholars of the world. He was a hard worker, a very personable individual. He was easy to work with. I have been surprised that one of our buildings hasn't been named for Dean Seashore."

In the ASHA Honors citation for Seashore, Johnson writes of his "progressive leadership, scientific shrewdness, broad sympathies, and personal encouragement" as an "extraordinary source of vision and resolve" for those working in the new field of speech correction.

LEADERSHIP CHANGES

Very early in his administration Johnson was faced with an almost complete change of personnel among the department heads and deans with whom the Program had carried on its work. In the first place there was the loss of Seashore. The Dean had given sustained leadership to interdepartmental cooperation from the Seashore-Orton-Mabie-Travis days to the time of his retirement, and then again when he came out of retirement to serve during the war years.

In a February 1949 memo Johnson, who always kept Seashore's portrait on his office wall, noted that the Dean's activities had extended to Speech, the College of Education, the Child Welfare Research Station, the Psychopathic Hospital, the Departments of Otolaryngology, Anatomy, Physiology, and Physics, and, finally, the School of Social Work, established that year with Wayne Vasey as director. (Vasey was succeeded in 1954 by Mark Hale, who was succeeded in 1962 by Frank Glick;) Eleanor K. Taylor was acting director twice in those years. Also new in the picture was Dr. R. R. Rembolt, of the Hospital School for Severely Handicapped Children, established in 1947.

There was also new leadership in older campus units that has been associated with the Program. Robert Sears resigned in 1949 as director of the Child Welfare Research Station and was succeeded in 1951 by Boyd McCandless. Beth Wellman had been acting director in the interim.

Dewey Stuit moved from Psychology to become acting dean in 1948, and dean, in 1949, of the College of Liberal Arts. He succeeded Earl McGrath, dean from 1945 to 1948, who had succeeded Harry K. Newburn, dean from 1941 to 1945. Newburn had succeeded George F. Kay, dean from 1918 to 1941, and a member of Iowa's remarkable pioneering trio: Seashore, Jessup, Kay.

In the Graduate College, Carlyle Jacobsen had served as dean from 1946 to 1948, succeeding Seashore and being succeeded by Harvey Davis, dean from 1948 to 1950. In 1950 Walter F. Loehwing succeeded Davis. Davis, who had carried the double responsibilities of the deanship and those of the newly created administrative post of provost, was then able to turn all of his attention to the latter.

THE NEED FOR A "CONSTRUCTIVE SOLUTION"

By 1949, the year of Seashore's death, there were eighty-nine undergraduate majors in the Program, forty-two M.A. candidates and nine post-M.A. students. That fall, 210 individuals were seen at the Speech Clinic, 128 from the schools of the community. Johnson wrote memo after memo to explain the administrative difficulties he faced. In May and again in November these memos were long and detailed. They were directed to the administration: Mabie, Spence, Provost Davis, and Dean Stuit. Wrote Johnson, "the marked and continuing growth of the Program in Speech Pathology and Audiology is serving to nourish certain old problems and to create new ones. Constructive solutions seem quite clearly indicated and I should like to recommend them to you."

He mentions the enrollment growth and the accompanying expansion of clinical case work "essential to professional training," then points out that the "medical faculty, particularly in otolaryngology and in the residential and outpatient services for handicapped children have been drawn increasingly into the Program as well as such outside agencies as the State Services for the Deaf, the State School for the Blind, and the department of public instruction. Along with these and other related developments has gone necessarily a very noticeable increase in the scope and complexity of the problems of administration."

He then suggests these changes: recognition of Speech Pathology and Audiology as a major, so that students will not have to choose Speech or Psychology; catalogue listing of the Program as a major; authority for the director of the clinic to appoint M.A. and Ph.D. committees; availability of general activities of both departments to all students so as not to break up the group; and clarification of administrative obligations and limitations. The budget, he noted, was then fifty-five percent from Speech, forty percent from Otolaryngology, and five percent from Psychology: "There is no rationality in that situation. Psychology used to carry the largest share."

"In consideration of this very important matter," he suggests,

> there should be a frank facing of the question of whether a separate budget should be assigned to the Speech Pathology and Audiology Program. At present I have to discharge considerable administrative responsibility, with no corresponding budgetary authority. Every staff member and assistant for whose work I am administratively responsible is budgetarily responsible to someone else. I find this

arrangement as difficult, frustrating, and embarrassing as any of you would and I am convinced that it is an unsound arrangement. I could operate much more efficiently if I had a budget covering secretarial assistance, office and clinical supplies, and basic laboratory equipment, and at least assistants and instructors, if not also part- and full-time ranking staff members, including myself, directly involved in the Program. Whatever may be done about this, it is essential that staff members be officially assigned to the Program and that my administrative obligations and limitations regarding them be clarified sufficiently for practical purposes.

In the May memo Johnson had also requested that he be allowed to add a new course called The Psychology of Speech and Hearing Disorders, which he would teach. It is needed, he wrote, "because so many speech pathology majors are not about to get into the clinical psychology courses."

Then he continued,

We need an established and recognized undergraduate curriculum. As it is now a major in Psychology is required to take experimental psychology and statistics. A major in Speech is required to take public speaking, public discussion and debate, dramatic interpretation, voice and phonetics. The Graduate programs vary too.

Next year no assistantships will be available in psychology so all must be in speech. . . . Psychologists are not available as needed for psychological tests in the clinic. The soundproof room, second floor center, used to be available for hearing testing and research in audiometry and experimental phonetics. Now it is used for studies in experimental psychology and for all practical purposes is no longer available to us. . . .

We need equipment. We need space. We would like all the barracks east of East Hall in which we now use four rooms; the veterans administration will vacate these barracks in June. We need space for the clinic "sometime" perhaps in the west wing of the East Hall ground floor.

SPACE PROBLEMS

The spaciousness which came with the move to East Hall in 1929 was now long gone, and the Program was faced with the problem of cramped quarters. At the beginning of the third period, the speech clinic was housed on the ground floor of the east wing of East Hall. Other parts of the Program were in four rooms of a barracks east of East Hall and in an area on the third floor, center section, of East Hall. All were crowded. Additional areas were shared with other departments, but these too were crowded because of the University's growth. The old sound-treated room in the northeast corner of the ground floor east section, for example, built with such joy by Metfessel, Lewis, Tiffin and others when the Program was young, was still used by both Psychology and the Program—but Psychology needed the room.

The same was true of the Psychology laboratory. "In these days," says Curtis *(1)*, speaking of the people in Psychology, "there was a very close working relationship and they were very gracious to us. But we simply needed more space and so did they."

It was about 1950, as Curtis recalls, that Strother and his colleagues at the University of Washington invited him to join them to build up their experimental phonetics program. Mabie, who as head of the Speech Department was now virtually the administrative head of the Program, asked Curtis what it would take to keep him at Iowa. Curtis replied: "Laboratory equipment and laboratory space including an anechoic chamber in which we could do some acoustic-phonetics kinds of research we were unable to do without such facilities." And so, Curtis continues, "Mabie said he would see what he could do. And it was then that the space of E-11 was given to us to fit out in any way we felt would make it usable as a laboratory." Curtis and the University architect, George Horner, collected ideas in visits to other installations, then proceeded to build. By 1952 the new laboratory was in full operation. It continued for the rest of the Program's days in East Hall, and always in E-11.

Lack of space was so much a problem that hearing testing of incoming University students was omitted altogether one semester in the 1950-51 academic year. Johnson, in an April 1951 memo to Dean Loehwing, explains that there simply was no place available and sufficiently quiet for the testing.

In this memo Johnson was stating the need for reconditioned quarters, apparently in the barracks, "in order to carry on the essential hearing testing of our own student body and to provide essential research and professional training facilities in connection with our graduate training and research program in audiology."

Reger and Curtis had both been involved in this, he noted. Then he added that the United States Children's Bureau, through the Reger program in SSCC, had approved more than $4,000 for equipment, and that the Bureau had increased its annual grant from $12,000 to $22,000 to support the training program in audiology.

Meanwhile, in the spring of 1951, when the Romance Language Department moved its language laboratory from East Hall, third floor center, to Schaeffer Hall, the Program was assigned the rooms thus vacated and immediately began remodeling there. Some of the larger spaces were cut up into small rooms for clinical and experimental uses. Sound-treated booths, eventually four in all, were installed. One room became a multipurpose area that served as a seminar room, classroom, small group meeting room, and listening laboratory. It was fitted with a special sound absorbing acoustic treatment on the walls, and was wired for group listening by both earphone and loudspeaker so it could be used in various types of perceptual experiments and also in experiments with group hearing testing procedures.

This area was in use by 1952. About the same time, the old brick house south of the zoology building on Dubuque Street—known as The Gables—was assigned to the Program as an annex. Additional space was also assigned in barracks east of East Hall, where three or four rooms had been used by the Program since 1947.

AT LAST, A COUNCIL

Early in 1951, a quarter century after Travis finished his postdoctoral training and officially assumed leadership of the Program, a Council on Speech Pathology and Audiology was created by action of the Graduate College. This gave the Program its first administrative framework.

Invitations to serve on the Council were issued by Dean Loehwing in the form of a memo March 29, 1951, addressed to Johnson and Spriestersbach of the Speech Clinic, Dr. Lierle, Dr. Rembolt, and Dean Stuit, all of whom agreed to serve. Carbons of the memo went to Spence, Mabie, and Provost Davis.

Dean Loehwing pointed out that the Council would be set up in the Graduate College. Its function, he explained, would be "primarily to expedite administration on the academic aspects of the students' majors in the fields of Speech Pathology and Audiology, and to represent the University in essential liaison relationships with public and private agencies concerned with the program."

The Council held its first meeting on May 26, 1951. It attended to necessary items of business, then took a little time to review the history of the preceding twenty-five years. And, though a span of twenty-five years may have skimped a bit on the beginnings of the beginnings, it was adequate to cover Travis's last year of postdoctoral training, his entire term as administrator, Strother's entire period, too, and four years of Johnson's—thus including the broader aspects of the entire story of the new discipline to date.

Johnson was named chairman of the Council, Spriestersbach, secretary; Dr. Lierle and Dr. Rembolt were the other appointed members; Dean Stuit and Dean Loehwing served *ex officio*.

Spriestersbach *(19)* recalls that his duties were something like those of a chief of staff, to use a military phrase. He handled a great deal of the day-to-day paper work, took on much of the academic advising in the Department, and conferred with Johnson once a day or so to talk over problems and projects. Spriestersbach remembers the arrangement as a pleasant one. He had become known for his ability at organizing—he had had his army training and a year in personnel work in industry before returning to Iowa for his Ph.D. And Johnson, he explains, "just didn't want to be bothered with details of running the office, moment to moment. And I remember how appreciative he was of being relieved of that kind of work. It's interesting. There were those who seemed to think there was some kind of magic in organizing, where, as far as I can see, there is nothing involved but just sheer figuring out when two should come after one."

So the Council was organized and work committees were set up. These included:

Professional Training, Spriestersbach, Curtis, Darley, Johnson, Schubert;

Research, Curtis, Darley, Johnson, Reger, Schubert, Sherman, Spriestersbach;

Audiology, Schubert, Curtis, Johnson, Keaster, Reger;

Clinical Practice, Darley, Johnson, Keaster, Sherman, Spriestersbach;

Professional Affairs, Keaster, Curtis, Darley;

Student Affairs, Spriestersbach;

Interagency Relationships, Darley, Johnson, Keaster;

Clinical Service Units, (chairmen). Dr. Lierle for Otolaryngology, Dr. Rembolt for State Services for Crippled Children, and Darley for the Speech Clinic.

Authority and Responsibility. Establishment of the Council had helped, but there were problems still, as Johnson wrote in a March 1952 memo to the members of that Council. He cited particularly the breakdown of communication in specific areas and the discrepancy between the authority he had and the responsibility he carried as Council chairman. He saw the need for a speech clinic supervisor. He even wondered if the situation might be improved if he were relieved of his administrative duties so he could use his "time and ability more effectively in teaching and research."

A Haphazard Shift. Then he goes on to say,

I feel that the recent heavy shift of the Program from psychology to speech and dramatic arts has been essentially haphazard, brought about by professionally irrelevant motivations, and that if the department of psychology or the department of speech and dramatic arts has benefited, or has not, this consequence has been a matter of chance. At the same time it is clear that the department of speech and dramatic arts has afforded the Program during a period of marked expansion, strong support and a congenial atmosphere.

Consequently, the department has a considerable vested interest in the Speech Pathology and Audiology Program and I think it would be desirable to keep the two closely associated.

THE COUNCIL ONE YEAR LATER

The problems of administration continued to be cited by Johnson. In his report of the first year's activities under the Council he notes that clinical services were provided through eight different departments, colleges, and agencies. Laboratories were in five departments in three colleges. The fourteen full-time staff workers (instructor to professor) were affiliated with eight departments or agencies and paid from six budgets; twenty-one part-time assistants and fellows were paid from five budgets; and one half-time and four full-time secretaries were paid from three budgets. Required courses were from eight different departments; four additional departments contributed electives. Some days he was heard to wonder aloud, in the face of an administrative decision, "which prayer rug to use."

Enrollment in September 1951, he reported, was 140 undergraduate and graduate majors. Many of these came from great distances, some from foreign countries, evidence of the Program's reputation. Speech examinations were given to 4,959 individuals, including University students; therapy was given to 325 in the spring semester of 1951, 126 in the summer session, and 342 in the fall semester. The spring and fall surveys of University students included 1,248 speech tests and 843 hearing tests.

He noted outside support from two sources, the Hill Family Foundation and the United States Children's Bureau. Support of the Hill Family Foundation, which was to continue through Johnson's life, and which grew in 1963 to include all of his academic enterprise, began in September 1951 with a $58,408 grant for two student projects and the publication (7) of a backlog of completed studies. The period of this grant was three years. The United States Children's Bureau had made a $20,000 grant in aid for the professional training program in audiology. This grant was administered by the Iowa State Services for Crippled Children.

TWO PROPOSALS

The University administration, concerned about the procedural problems of the Program, in 1952 discussed two proposals for something more than the Council but less than a Department. Neither proposal was adopted, but both seem to have contributed to the ongoing discussion of autonomy.

A Center. The first of these two proposals would have established a Speech Pathology and Audiology Center which would have been an interdepartmental agency to facilitate and coordinate studies in the "analysis and treatment of speech and hearing difficulties." It would have been supported jointly by the College of Liberal Arts, the Graduate College, the College of Medicine, foundation grants, and funds from government agencies.

The Center would be responsible to a committee consisting of the deans of the colleges in which it was budgeted and the dean of the Graduate College. The dean of the college in which the major portion of the program was located would be chairman. The committee would be responsible to the provost.

Operating policy and practice would be guided by an administrative committee of representatives from cooperating departments, bureaus, and clinics, to be appointed by the deans' committee. Suggested membership included Mabie, Arthur Benton of Psychology, James Stroud of Psychology and Education, Curtis, Dr. Lierle, Dr. Raymond Rembolt, then director of State Services for Crippled Children, Vasey of the School of Social Work, and McCandless of Child Welfare. The proposed staff would be Johnson as director, Spriestersbach as associate director, and Schubert as a staff member.

The Center would not, the proposal said, grant degrees; enrollment would be in Speech in the College of Liberal Arts for undergraduates, and in the Graduate College in Speech, Psychology, or Education for graduate students. The Speech Clinic would be a division of the Department of Speech.

A Unit in the School of Speech. The second proposal was made by Mabie at a staff meeting of the Speech Department, then officially the Department of Speech and Dramatic Arts, during the summer of 1952. This proposal, tentatively agreed upon by the faculty, would have created a Department of Speech Pathology and Audiology within a *school* of speech. Mabie had outlined several possibilities, in all of which Speech Pathology and Audiology was treated as an autonomous entity, equal in status to the other Department divisions.

Johnson protested in a memo to Dean Stuit, with carbons to Mabie and Dean Loehwing. He pointed out that since 1949 he had worked for some kind of autonomy, and had objected to "absorption within the department of speech and dramatic arts of the traditionally interdepartmental Speech Pathology and Audiology Program."

Then he goes on to say that if the Program were to become part of the Speech Department, this arrangement would amount to a

radical departure from the long established and previously unchallenged policy of guarding against the annexation of the Program by any single established department. This policy has been adhered to since it was initiated more than a quarter of a century ago

. . . since interdepartmental relationships under which the traditional Seashore policy operated no longer exist, I am convinced that the interests of all concerned are to be served best by granting to the speech pathology and audiology group an individual status in which it will have the freedom necessary to grow internally and to develop its own functional relations to various other departments, colleges, and agencies in ways that are professionally logical and most fruitful.

That status would come eventually, but not during Johnson's administration.

CHANGES REFLECTED IN CATALOGUE PAGES

University catalogue listings for the Program in this period continue for the first two years with little change. They are, as before, in Speech and Psychology. They are not grouped in Speech, but they are in Psychology (as they have been since 1946), under "Speech Pathology and Hearing Conservation." Three major changes come in the third year, in catalogue No. 1950, for 1949-50. The heading in Psychology becomes "Speech Pathology and Audiology," the book's index carries a "speech pathology and audiology" entry (the first time the Program's course work had been indexed), and the Psychology test includes a line referring to the "complete listing" in speech.

In catalogue No. 1951, for 1950-51, Speech Department listings are reorganized into six major sections. The second of these is headed "Phonetics and Speech Laboratory, James F. Curtis, advisor," the fifth is headed "Speech Pathology & Audiology, Wendell Johnson, advisor." Finally, and almost as an addendum to the department listings but not identified as part of those listings, is a section headed "Speech Pathology and Audiology, Wendell Johnson, Director of the Speech Clinic, Room E-14, East Hall." This was a year before the Council, six years before the Department, yet the printing type used for the heading is the same size and kind as that used for department headings. The page overlines, "Speech Pathology and Audiology," also are in "department" style. Progress, it seems, was being made in some ways, even if not officially.

Text, in this unusual addendum, filled three columns with general information and course descriptions. Students planning to major in speech pathology and audiology are advised to consult the director of the Speech Clinic before registering, and are told that they may major in speech pathology but not in audiology for the B.A., but may major in either of those areas, or may combine them, for the M.A. and the Ph.D. degrees. All three degrees

are granted through the Departments of Speech and Psychology, but candidates major in Speech Pathology and Audiology, not in the departments as such. . . . Undue specialization at the B.A. level is discouraged. . . . Any student who plans to work in the public schools must take courses in education leading to the required certification for teaching. . . . Candidates for the M.A. degree are required to present a minimum of 38 semester hours of approved course work beyond the B.A. degree [with writing of thesis optional]. . . . Candidates for the Ph.D. degree are required to take either Foundations of Measurement . . . or Advanced Statistical Methods. . . .

(It is just possible that this Ph.D. requirement is related to some of the problems Johnson mentioned on occasion, problems that resulted from the heavy emphasis on statistics in Psychology and the relatively light emphasis on that area in Speech.)

Course listings reflect something of the interdepartmental nature of the Program. Several courses have double or triple listing, usually in Speech and/or Psychology and the Program. The ones most consistently listed in this way were Curtis's phonetics and speech laboratory courses and Johnson's general semantics course. Since that first listing in the 1950-51 catalogue, the Speech Department has carried the laboratory in its offerings every year to the present (1968), its eighteenth consecutive listing.

The Council. Finally, in catalogue No. 1952, for the year 1951-52, the Council appears in print. Section V of the Speech Department listings is headed "Speech Pathology and Audiology"; Chairman of the University Council on Speech Pathology and Audiology, Wendell Johnson; Administrative Assistant, D. C. Spriestersbach." Below that, in the order of their listing, are courses taught by Sherman, Johnson, Spriestersbach, Darley, Keaster, Reger, and Schubert. Curtis is not included here, but in the Speech Laboratory section. As in the preceding year, there is the addendum at the end of the Department's listing. This time it is headed "Speech Pathology and Audiology, Programs of Study," and it fills two and a half pages. Beginning in 1953 the Program advanced one more step toward official recognition: its clinical work was cited in the catalogue section on research and service units.

In the catalogue for 1954-55 comes the final major catalogue change in the period. For the first time since the beginning of the Program, its courses are not listed in Psychology, they are listed only in Speech.

CURRICULUM DEVELOPMENT

Catalogue listings for 1955, the final year of this period, suggest something of the curriculum development that had taken place. It is to be recalled that when this period began in 1947, Johnson and Curtis were the only faculty members working full time in the Program. Excerpts from Sections II and

V of the Speech Department's listings for that final year, from catalogue No. 1955, follow.

Section II: Phonetics and Speech Laboratory, James F. Curtis, Professor in charge, office C307 East Hall. Voice and Phonetics, Curtis; Voice and Speech Development, Lynch; Principles of Laboratory Instrumentation, Curtis; Experimentation, Curtis; Experimental Phonetics (two-course sequence), Curtis; Research in Experimental Phonetics [no instructor listed], credits arranged.

Section V: Speech Pathology and Audiology, Chairman of the Council, Wendell Johnson; Administrative Assistant, D. C. Spriestersbach. Individual Instruction in the Speech Clinic, Darley and Clinic staff; Methods in Public School Speech Correction, Sherman; General Semantics, Johnson; Introduction to Speech Pathology and Audiology, Spriestersbach; Fundamentals of Hearing, Schubert; Problems in Speech Pathology and Audiology, Staff; Diagnosis and Appraisal in Speech Pathology, Darley; Voice and Articulation Disorders, Sherman; Stuttering: Research and Theory, Johnson; Organic Disorders of Speech I, Darley; Organic Disorders of Speech II, Spriestersbach; Communication Problems of the Hard of Hearing, Parker; Measurement of Hearing Loss, Parker; Seminar, Speech Pathology and Audiology I, Staff; Seminar, Speech Pathology and Audiology II, Staff; Advanced Audiometry, Reger; Experimental Audiology I, Testing and Measurement in Audition, Schubert; Experimental Audiology II, Problems in Clinical Diagnosis, Schubert; Experimental Audiology III, Electrophysiology in Audition, Schubert; Advanced Clinical Practice in Speech Pathology and Audiology, Staff; Research in Speech Pathology and Audiology, Staff; Internship in Speech Pathology, Staff; Internship in Audiology, Staff; Seminar, Research Design in Speech and Hearing, Sherman [this included new technique in scaling as noted below].

PSYCHOSOCIAL ORIENTATION

Throughout the years of this period, Johnson pioneered in developing a psychosocial approach to the study of speech problems, specifically stuttering, and particularly in Onset Studies II and III (*8*, pp. 8-10 and *passim*) which had grown out of his own earlier research, Onset Study I, undertaken in the years 1934 to 1940. Study II, 1948 to 1952, centered in Darley's Ph.D. research; Study III involved the work of others and was ongoing at the end of the period.

Johnson encouraged the new approach in the research of others when their aim, like his, was to understand not only the speech handicap as such but also the context in which it had become a problem of personal interaction and reaction for both speaker and listener. On occasion he told his classes that stuttering, for example, begins in the ear of the speaker's mother and usually when the speaker is a child of about three.

Some years later, in answer to a request to evaluate his work in speech pathology and audiology, Johnson *(3)* said he regarded the Onset Studies as the "most important research" he had done. This research involves, he explained, "a really major departure not only from previous theories of stuttering presented by other writers but also from my own previously published thinking."

One notable program soon to grow out of the new psychosocial approach was Spriestersbach's research in problems of cleft lip and palate. Although there are all sorts of antecedents, Spriestersbach *(19)* says he can "pinpoint almost to the day" the beginning of this. He was walking with Johnson and others from East Hall for a seminar. This was in the early fifties when he had just taken over the coursework in organic speech disorders. Johnson

> got to talking about Darley's work and the relationships that this whole technique had to various problems in the area, when he turned to me and said, "What do you know about the impact of a cleft upon youngsters?" Well, of course, I hadn't any clinical experience to fall back on and obviously there wasn't anything in the literature. I don't know that we pursued it much that day. He didn't press me. But I didn't forget it. It started some thinking on my part: why not try to use a design something like the Onset Studies, the coded questionnaire and the whole technique.

And so he devised his plan. The questionnaire included some items from Darley's, coded to show the relation. Then he tried to get a grant to support the project. He was turned down twice, but the third time was successful. And so it was that in 1955, the closing year of the Johnson period, he began his project. (Because of the double Iowa connection, it is interesting to note that in these years he was becoming active in the American Association of Cleft Palate Prostheses which had been organized in 1934 by Iowa's Herbert Koepp-Baker, Ph.D. 1938. Later the organization became the American Cleft Palate Association, and Spriestersbach was its president in 1961-62.)

STUTTERING RESEARCH AND THEORY

In a brief review of his work with stuttering in this period, Johnson *(5)* later explained that the purpose of his clinical work then was to try to modify "the stuttering reactions in the direction of encouraging the speaker to perform them more simply, with minimal muscular effort, and with minimal inhibition, or maximal spontaneity," an emphasis that developed from his earlier research into the nature of stuttering (see Chapter 5). In 1953 he began a long-term study to evaluate stuttering therapy in the Speech Clinic, a study supported continuously from 1953 to the time of his death by the Louis W. and Maud Hill Family Foundation, and in the late fifties by other agencies as well. Many students did research in stuttering in their graduate programs. In a 1962 report of the Department to the administration, the statement is made that the research output in the area of stuttering is "unquestionably larger than that of any other university."

Thirty Years of Research. Toward the end of the third period Johnson edited, with the assistance of Ralph R. Leutenegger (Iowa Ph.D., 1953, later at Michigan State University, then at the University of Wisconsin, Milwaukee) a book called *Stuttering in Children and Adults (7),* which he described as a record of thirty years of research at The University of Iowa. The volume, copyrighted in 1955, is dedicated to Travis, Mabie, Stoddard, and the memory of Seashore.

Through the book Johnson has noted trends and changes which are of historical interest, among them these:

> In recent years all the ranking members of the Speech Pathology and Audiology staff at Iowa (James Curtis, Frederic L. Darley, Charles D. Parker, Scott N. Reger, Dorothy Sherman, Earl Schubert, D. C. Spriestersbach, Jacqueline Keaster, now on the staff of the Childrens Hospital in Los Angeles, and myself) have worked as a research team in the stuttering area as well as in other areas of the general program. . . . [pp. IX, X]
>
> Chapters of Part II contain the sum and substance of Iowa research findings to date (a portion published in 1942) with respect to the onset and early development of stuttering. . . . [p. 36]
>
> The first systematic and comprehensive study of the fluency dimension of children's speech was made by Davis, who reported her findings in the *Journal of Speech Disorders* in 1939. Subsequent investigations were done by Branscom, Hughes, and Oxtoby . . . related studies were by Egland, Mann, and Johnson. . . . In Part III the data from these six investigations provide . . . a generally full account of Iowa research so far completed on nonfluency in the speech of young children. . . . [p. 156]
>
> In 1933 the editor published in the *Quarterly Journal of Speech* an analysis of a single occurrence of stuttering, and as it turned out the chief implication of this analysis was that what we think of as stuttering reduces . . . to stutterings—and that stutterings can be counted. The first subsequent experimental study in which they were counted was done in 1933 by M. D. Steer as his master's thesis at Iowa. Since then variations in the amount of stuttering have been investigated with ever increasing procedural refinement and theoretical sophistication . . . studies that have been done in this phase of the research program . . . cover a span of twenty years. . . . Some of the more recent studies are impressively different from the early ones so far as methodology is concerned, but the early ones are included not only because some of the findings they yielded are of value in themselves, but also because

these pioneer studies are of considerable historical interest. . . . [p. 198]

The dominant traditional view of human behavior has been that structure determines function . . . [a] view . . . reflected in the beginning phases of the Iowa stuttering research program. Several years of investigative experience resulted in a shift to different emphases, however, and the data presented in Chapters 30 and 31 intimate the reason for this. . . . [p. 360]

The first graduate theses at the University of Iowa that were concerned exclusively with stuttering were written under the supervision of the late Professor John Madison Fletcher in . . . 1924 . . . by Marion McKenzie Font and Marion Brehm Hebenstreit. The third thesis in the Iowa stuttering research program was that of Bryng Bryngelson, directed by Professor Lee Edward Travis in 1926. These first three dissertations, together with two other early M.A. theses by Lois Hickman Adams and S. Spencer Shaw, are here published for the first time. They are presented in the form of brief abstracts. As the work of pioneers, indicative of the nature of certain early stirrings in stuttering research, they are to be entered most appropriately in the record. . . . [p. 388]

All who do research on stuttering are motivated, certainly, by the great hope that their efforts will lead to sound principles and effective procedures of prevention and of retraining. The chapters which comprise this final section modestly represent that hope. . . . Finally, some eighteen years ago the editor set down certain notions about stuttering therapy which seemed to him to recommend themselves, and in the concluding chapter of this volume they appear for the first time in published form. *This chapter is believed to have been the first statement on the treatment of stuttering written from a semantic point of view,* and it is chiefly on this account that it makes such claim on the reader's attention as it may properly presume to make. . . . [p. 404, italics ours]

Theses and Publications. A bibliography of Iowa studies in stuttering through 1954, included as an appendix, lists 101 M.A. theses, 51 Ph.D. dissertations, and 266 publications.

Speech Science

With the new laboratory equipment, the laboratory space in E-11 East Hall, and the anechoic chamber he had obtained from Mabie in 1950-51, Curtis proceeded to develop the curriculum in speech science in ways not possible without these. He worked with students not only in Speech Pathology and Audiology but also with those in the Department of Speech and Dramatic Arts. That Department listed the laboratory as a major curriculum unit in the University catalogue for 1950-51, catalogue No. 1951, and has continued to do so since, making the listing for 1968, the final year included in the present writing, the eighteenth in that long series.

Within the Program, speech science became increasingly important as the faculty came more and more to see it as the fundamental curriculum on which, ideally, specialization should rest. In other words, the undergraduate curriculum should be broad and basic; specialization should come at the graduate level.

This point of view was committed to print in a tentative sort of way in catalogue No. 1951 in the notation that undue specialization at the B.A. level was "discouraged." To hold this point of view was in itself to pioneer, because at that time speech pathology and audiology was very new in the world of academe. It was included in the curriculum of only a limited number of universities and colleges, and the vocational B.A., so to speak, was generally considered standard in terms of preparation for professional work in the field.

Curtis says there were many faculty discussions of the matter. And so the movement away from the terminal B.A. continued to be encouraged throughout the period, foreshadowing changes that would come not only at Iowa but within the profession at large in the sixties.

THE SCALING OF SEVERITY

Lewis made a public presentation of his pioneering work in the psychological scaling of the severity of speech disorders, in this case stuttering, at the 1950 convention of the American Speech and Hearing Association in session in Columbus, Ohio. This was at a section on research approaches to stuttering, chaired by Lewis's former student at Iowa, John Black. George Wischner, another Iowan but of a slightly later time (Black's Ph.D. was 1935, Wischner's, 1947), appeared at the same session. Then, in 1951, Lewis and Sherman presented this material and the results of additional work in an article in the December issue of the *Journal of Speech and Hearing Disorders (11).* This was the first publication anywhere of the basic methodology used to obtain psychologically scaled samples of stuttered speech. Severity was measured in terms of difficulty at the moment rather than in terms of moments per unit of time. It was demonstrated, the authors wrote, that by the use of the scaling method of equal appearing intervals, severity of the auditory characteristics of stuttering "can be reliably measured solely on the basis of what is heard."

BACKWARD PLAY

About this time Sherman began working on the problem of irrelevant cues in speech samples which were being used in the study of voice quality. By the academic year 1953-54 she had developed and had demonstrated the usefulness of a technique she called backward play. She had discovered that when recorded speech samples were played backward, the judges who were evaluating them were able to attend to voice quality as such and were not distracted by the meaning or other irrelevancies. This research technique has come to be used widely throughout the country.

AUDIOLOGY WITHIN THE COUNCIL

With Schubert a member of the faculty, the Council could begin to develop its own program in audiology and thus lean less heavily than it had for so many years on the Department of Otolaryngology and Maxillofacial Surgery. Schubert came in 1951, and it was during that academic year that the Council had a visit from a man who was then in a signal corps laboratory in New Jersey, a man by the name of Paul Griffith—the same Paul Griffith who years before had succeeded Ted Hunter as designer and builder of instruments for Travis and others, including Curtis and Knott, in the very early days of the Program.

The Signal Corps was interested in certain problems of speech research. Griffith had come, as Curtis recalls, to see

whether we would be interested in undertaking a signal corps contract to do some research. And so we talked over ideas. Eventually we agreed to make an investigation of the problems of sidetone. This became known as the sidetone project. There was a substantial amount of interest in this kind of thing at the time. John Black and his group at Ohio State were involved from the standpoint of navy aviation. And he also had a project at Pensacola, supported by the navy. They were working on somewhat similar kinds of problems, of the way in which a person's hearing of himself monitors his speech. About this time [Bernard S.] Lee [then with the Signal Corps Engineering Laboratories, Fort Monmouth, New Jersey] had stumbled onto the phenomenon of speech disruption by delayed sidetone. People studying stuttering were interested in this effect which Lee called artificial stuttering although I think it would be generally agreed that this was not genuine stuttering at all. With all of this going on there was general interest in this whole process of self-hearing and its effect on speech and speech communication.

Now the signal corps was interested in this from a somewhat practical point of view since military communication is sometimes carried on under very difficult conditions, often times with tremendously high levels of noise, which would affect the way one hears himself. They were interested not only from a practical point of view however, but also from the viewpoint of basic research by which the whole process would be better understood. And so this was the kind of problem we studied, the auditory feedback problem; we looked at all the variables involved in this; we tried to determine as much as we possibly could what the physical pathways were, what kind of signal actually arrived at the ear, how and how much the signal was changed.

Of the two major pathways of sound, the airborne and the tissue-conducted, very little was known then about the latter. To learn more about the actual physical nature of the vibrations that travel through the tissues and arrive at the cochlea turned out to be a very difficult problem, technically. We tried to do a good deal of work on that. We were not very successful. John Dolch [Iowa Ph.D., 1953] did some of the work on this that was more definitive than anybody else's I would say. But I don't know that we have good definitive answers still.

There was not much publication of our work beyond the Signal Corps report *(16)*. People were not as pleased as they might have been with the kind of data they were getting. They wanted to improve and revise their techniques so they could get better data. None of us were as happy with the progress of the project as we would like to have been but I think it was a mistake that more was not published. Even if you haven't the final definitive answer doesn't mean that what you have found isn't important.

The people most involved were Schubert, Dolch, Richard Voots (Iowa Ph.D. 1955), Chester Atkinson, and Robert Seibel. Voots, later to join the faculty, was a doctoral candidate working gradually toward his degree but spending a substantial part of his time as an electronics technician. Seibel, a doctoral candidate in Psychology, and Atkinson, an Ohio State Ph.D. under Black, were brought in on the project as research associates.

"We had to devise much of our own instrumentation," Curtis explains, "and this was done in the East Hall laboratory. We developed an audiospectrometer, for example, an instrument for making spectroanalyses of speech more or less continuously and instantaneously as people talked. Voots worked on this a good deal. There were similar instruments but ours was somewhat different."

The final report was written in 1954. Sidetone research continued at Iowa but with less emphasis than during the project years.

A NEW VENTURE IN AUDIOMETRY

It was during approximately the same time as the sidetone project, early in the Johnson period, that Reger entered into a national and international adventure with the Bekesy audiometer. While, strictly speaking, this may not be part of the history of the Iowa Program in Speech Pathology and Audiology, it seems too closely related to be overlooked.

Georg von Bekesy, writing in *Acta Laryngologica* in 1947, described an audiometer he had designed and was then using in Sweden's Karolinska Institute, where he was working at the time. Reger read the article.

"I realized," Reger *(15)* explains,

that here was something different and probably superior to other testing procedures. There was just this one machine—no place in the world where I could buy one—so I built one.

Of course I wrote Professor Bekesy first to see if he would give me patent rights. And he was very nice. He said, "Well, go ahead and make six or eight or ten, and let's see if people want these things." I still have his letter. So we worked out an agreement and I made quite a few audiometers, and it really reached a point where I had to decide whether I was going to be a manufacturer or a university professor. I like teaching and research and so on. So I stopped building audiometers. I haven't made one for years.

Not long before he stopped a Japanese physician was studying with him, using one of his audiometers. The physician asked if Reger would build him one. Reger would, and did, and shipped it to him in Japan after he had returned there. Many years later when he was in Japan for this physician's celebration of his twentieth anniversary in practice, Reger discovered, to his considerable surprise and pleasure, that his had been the first Bekesy audiometer in the orient. So now he had a first on two continents, a first in America, then a first in Asia!

(As of 1968 Reger was writing a manual on Bekesy audiometry, to be dedicated to Bekesy, whom he had come to know well over the years and whose work was cited in an ASHA Honors award in 1966. Reger continued to experiment in his laboratory with a Bekesy audiometer of his own building, one with an amazing array of additions and changes to suit his needs. "When I wish that I could make a certain kind of measurement with it, I build it," he explains. He thinks he may be giving some papers on new things he has been able to find out about hearing because he could make his audiometer "do new tricks.")

REUNION

Related to the work in stuttering were two "reunions" in the early fifties when Lee Travis and his students from the Program's very early days gathered to talk about the theories each had since developed about stuttering.[3] The first gathering was in 1950 at the convention of the American Speech and Hearing Association in Columbus. Carl Ritzman of the University of Oklahoma, Iowa M.A. 1935, Ph.D. 1941, was section chairman. The subject was "Stuttering Twenty Years Later." The speakers were Bryng Bryngelson of the University of Minnesota, Charles Van Riper of the University of Western Michigan, Johnson of The University of Iowa, and Travis of the University of Southern California.

The second gathering was in Iowa City in 1952 when Travis, Van Riper,

Johnson, and Knott, now of Psychiatry at Iowa, were the speakers. This occasion was a summer conference called "Twenty-five Years of Stuttering Research and its Clinical Application." Spriestersbach served as chairman, presiding at the three sessions. Tape recordings of these sessions, now in the Johnson collection in University archives, indicate that it was a lively affair, with plenty of give and take of ideas, perhaps in the challenge everything spirit associated with the Travis days. Unfortunately lacking from the archival record, either on tape or in manuscript, is the Mabie luncheon address which Travis (23) remembers as a masterpiece. It was witty, graceful, and perceptive. It also was unusually complete for, it seems, Mabie had not missed much down through the years, and on this occasion wrapped up the history of the Program as neatly as anyone ever had.

After the final session of the conference, which was a bristling discussion session on a Saturday morning, Travis recalls that he and the other three participants finally "came up with the thought that stuttering is like a pie of about eight pieces. And we named the pieces. And one of these was Johnson's semantogenics. But there were other pieces too. And Johnson agreed that there were." Then Travis explained that he had talked about the semantogencis theory with Johnson many times and that "I had told him that my quarrel was that the theory doesn't go far enough. The stutterer does not introject only the fact that he is a stutterer, that he is diagnosed as a stutterer. He introjects also the rejection of him."

When Travis invited contributions for his magnum opus, *Handbook of Speech Pathology (24)*, which he published in 1957 (and in 1968 was revising), he chose to include work of Iowa colleagues in each section. On stuttering he in a measure "replayed" the Iowa conference with articles by Johnson, Van Riper, and himself. Knott was there too, his theories included in the papers of the others. He did not appear as an author because by then he had moved completely into the field of electroencephalography and quite out of the area of speech disorders.

THE TAPE RECORDER

No recital of the history of Johnson's work with stuttering in this period would be complete without a word about the tape recorder, an instrument which he began to use in more or less traditional ways in 1952, but with which he experimented from then on, finding new services it could render, and eventually bringing it into the counseling situation as a "revising machine." In a taped lecture in the introduction to speech pathology and audiology course in June 1964 he explained,

> I have been tape recording nearly everything that I have done in the classroom or the clinic for about the last 12 years. It has been a source of amazement to me that people who work in our field, or teachers,

are so reluctant to use a tape recorder. This is a very powerful instrument. What for?

I have some uses that are rather obvious. [You would record] for anyone who couldn't come and who would want later to hear the lecture. You can lend the tapes. . . . I began using it to study my voice, then what I was saying. And I was simply amazed at what I heard.

The main reason is that the tape recorder is a very powerful instrument in connection with the general task of trying to improve speech of any person. There's simply nothing that can substitute for a machine like this that enables him to be able to listen to his own speech. The effect is always powerful. I think it is so powerful that I really believe that the single most effective thing we could do to improve the American education at all levels would be to put a tape-recorder in every classroom. . . .You wouldn't have to tell the teacher what to listen for. . . .I have found that you don't need to do this. [The listener] hears everything you do and he is just as appalled by it as you are and he corrects it without your telling him to. . . .

You will react to listening to your own tape in various ways. . . .Some of you, to begin with, will say, "Oh, that can't be me," and you'll reject it. Part of the reason for this is that you hear yourself . . . as others hear you, by airborne sound, whereas you normally hear yourself by bone and air. . . .But beyond that, many people reject what they hear on the tape because of what they hear themselves saying. . . .

I think what you are going to hear at first mainly is the tone. I was appalled by the tone. . . .I have developed, I think, a better tone . . . not so much like a county attorney. . . .And I have developed a counseling method in which I use the tape by having the counselee listen to it. You see, the tape-recorder is really a revising machine. It helps the counselee literally to revise himself out of his problem. [The tape for this lecture is in Department files.]

THE SUMMER RESIDENTIAL CLINIC

The Summer Residential Clinic was continuing through this period, growing and changing in structure and program to meet new needs as they arose. Mrs. Earl Schubert, in her report for 1948 when she was finishing her third summer as housemother, presented a picture of improvement and progress.[4] She mentioned, for example, that the position of Director of Dormitories had been created in 1947, and that Hildred Schuell was the first to hold it; that dormitory clinicians and a full-time nurse were added in 1948; and that the staff also included a recreation director.

She felt it had been particularly helpful to have a physician as director of the Clinic. She was referring, of course, to Dr. Brown, whose responsibilities for all outpatient work included the Summer Clinic. When he resigned in 1949, his duties as director of that Clinic were taken over by

Darley, who served in that position from 1950 until 1961. Parley Newman was supervisor of the dormitories in 1952, Paul Jensen in 1953, Maryjane Rees in 1954. All subsequently earned the Ph.D. degree at Iowa.

SPEECH CORRECTION IN STATE INSTITUTIONS

Another activity beyond student work in classrooms and laboratories centered in speech and hearing surveys and therapy programs of the kind mentioned in a 1942 position paper written by Fairbanks. He suggested that the Speech Clinic had a service obligation to the children in state institutions and schools, but his idea apparently was not implemented until the late forties and early fifties under Darley's leadership. (Children's institutions under the Iowa State Board of Control in 1968 were the State Juvenile Home in Toledo, the Glenwood State School in Glenwood, the Woodward State Hospital and School in Woodward, the State Training School for Girls at Mitchellville, the State Training School for Boys at Eldora, and the Iowa Annie Wittenmeyer Home in Davenport; and under the Iowa State Board of Regents—which in 1942 was called the Iowa State Board of Education—were the Iowa School for the Blind at Vinton and the Iowa School for the Deaf at Council Bluffs.)

Darley, in a December 1950 memo to Johnson, refers to student internships of previous years at both Vinton and Council Bluffs, then goes on to report results of the speech and hearing survey which thirty of his students, in his course in introduction to clinical practice, had made in November 1949 at Vinton. This survey was followed in the spring of 1950 by a speech correction program directed by Andrew Bodnar, a student intern who was earning credit toward his M.A. degree (1950) and who was supported jointly by the school and the Johnson County Society for Crippled Children and Adults. Bodnar, at the end of his internship, was employed as a full-time staff member at the school.

The purpose of the Darley memo was to suggest a program of testing and internships for the several state schools. Darley refers to conversations and correspondence with various officers of those schools and with Lowell B. Schenke, then psychologist, later director of psychological services, of the Board of Control.

Later that December, soon after the Darley memo was written, the Board of Control decided to provide funds for a speech survey and the services of an intern at five of their six institutions, omitting the Wittenmeyer Home. This omission may have been only a typographical error because Schenke, in January 1951, mentions the Darley plan for the *six* institutions and, in fact, Darley reports on a January 1951 speech survey at the Wittenmeyer Home. Barbara Stansell later served as the first intern there.

A survey was made at Toledo in 1951, and the next year Robert Lee

Rosenbaum became the intern there, earning credit toward his 1953 M.A. degree. Schenke subsequently brought Rosenbaum's report to the attention of the Board of Control in what seems to have been a move to inform the Board of certain problems in the Home. Schenke had mentioned these in explaining the difficulties he faced before he gained acceptance for himself and his work. Discipline at the Home was very strict. He found it was not unusual for children to be punished because they did not speak plainly. ("They're just showing off," one staff member explained.) By the end of his internship Rosenbaum faced at least one new problem: children feigned speech disorders to have an excuse to come to talk with him.

There are indications, from the records available, that both the speech surveys and the internships continued for some time, but apparently not on a regular schedule. A second survey of the Wittenmeyer Home is mentioned in 1954. The time came when surveys were made only if an intern was available to do follow-up work, which meant there were delays. As Darley pointed out, however, a survey without a follow-up could be less than helpful to both the children and the institution.

Some schools later continued in one way or another to give attention to the speech and hearing problems of their children. Some sent children to the summer residential clinic. And some did relatively little. But, overall, the project was regarded as having very positive results. The most active programs were at the School for the Blind, the Annie Wittenmeyer Home, the Woodward State Hospital and School, and the School for the Deaf.

THE SCHOOL FOR THE DEAF

The Iowa Program, and later the Council, at the time, Curtis recalls, had its most formal understandings with the School for the Deaf. These began about 1950 when Josephine Carr (Iowa M.A. 1951) was at the School as the principal of what was called the lower division. Before she finished her degree, and afterward, several students in the Program spent a semester, in one case a year, at the School learning about working with deaf children and also providing some services and doing some research studies on that population with respect to speech and hearing problems. For the most part, these students were working toward master's degrees, and master's theses resulted from the work they did.

Johnson, Reger, and Keaster had a good deal of interest in this. Related theses were done largely under Keaster's direction. The next development in relations between the School and the Council was to come after the close of the Johnson period.

A footnote might be added here. In a 1953 issue of the Iowa Speech and Hearing Association's *Iowa Therapist,* an item tells that the audiometer used in the beginning of the Program at the School for the Deaf was built by Ross Weaver in Reger's laboratory. Mention is also made in a later issue of the research done by Reger and his Japanese friend at the School.

STATE AND NATIONAL ACTIVITIES

During the Johnson period, faculty members were leaders in professional projects and activities at both the state and the national levels. At the beginning of the period these were a continuation, in spirit, if not in specifics, of those that went before; they proceed through the period as an integral part of the work load.

Iowa faculty members and people who had been trained in the Iowa Program gave leadership, for example, to the establishment of the Iowa Speech Correction Association in Old Capitol on the Iowa campus October 17, 1947. Curtis was elected president; Velma Bissell Hiser (Iowa M.A. 1938), of Grinnell College, vice-president; Marceline Smith, of the special education division of the State Department of Public Instruction, secretary-treasurer; and Josephine Simonson, of the Iowa State Teachers College (now University of Northern Iowa) English and Speech Department, editor of publications. The Iowa leadership continued from that time on.

Among those on the program the day of the organization meeting were: Mabie; Sherman, then in speech correction work in the Des Moines public schools; Mrs. Dorothy Phillips of the Iowa Society for Crippled Children and Adults, who had worked with Strother and his colleagues in the pioneering projects that fed into the Hospital School; and Dr. Ernest Fossum (Iowa M.A. 1933, Ph.D. 1941) of the ISTC Speech Clinic.

According to the Association records, the twenty-three charter members, that is, those who paid the one dollar membership fee at that time, included five who then were or later would be members or affiliates of the Iowa faculty: Curtis, Johnson, Keaster, Bette Spriestersbach, and Sherman.

The name of the Association was changed, on a motion by Johnson and seconded by Keaster at the May 1950 annual meeting, to be effective January 1952. The new name, Iowa Speech and Hearing Association, has been in use ever since.

Iowa was the fifth state in the nation to have a speech correction association *(13)*. The first ten were Indiana and Utah in 1937, Michigan and Wisconsin in 1939, Iowa in 1947, Oregon in 1949, California and Connecticut in 1950, and Colorado in 1951.

Iowa, The Association, and Certification

With Curtis as president, the new Association concerned itself almost immediately with the problem of certifying people in the field. And, as Curtis recalls, "it was a problem. That was the beginning of our work on it. This continued for several years, one way or another, with the group in the University taking leadership. We had very fine backing from our own College of Education and Dean E. T. Peterson. We eventually got the job done."

Soon after World War II an endorsement in speech correction was officially adopted as part of the certification regulations for teachers in the state of Iowa, which meant that a person with this endorsement was recognized as qualified in this field to do work in the public schools. The endorsement required, first of all, Curtis explains,

> that a person be a certified teacher, that is, meet all the requirements for certification as a teacher in elementary or secondary school or both, and that meant taking a tremendous amount of work that many of us felt was not relevant to remedial speech work.
>
> And secondly, the amount of actually relevant coursework and experience required for this endorsement was so minimal as to be nearly meaningless. It was the kind of work that a person could accomplish in a summer or, at most, a semester, three courses at the most, of really relevant information. So these requirements meant that people would be trained adequately as teachers but completely inadequately in the special area which by this time had far advanced beyond the point where one could encompass the knowledge in that short a period. And so we thought that these were completely inadequate kinds of requirements.

A certain man in the State Department of Public Instruction who had helped draw up the requirements insisted that they had been developed after looking at the requirements in all states that had this kind of requirement. "Our point was," Curtis continues,

> that he had never consulted with us and we were the experts in the field in the state of Iowa. He had never come to us even for a question or to look over what was being proposed. These requirements were past history, not looking forward to what ought to be. We really reached an impasse with him.
>
> Finally we were able to get him and some of the other people from the State Department to sit down around a table with us and we had Dean Peterson and one or two others from the College of Education to sit down with us. [This was in the winter of 1949.] We had people from the state department and I think Jessie Parker (State Superintendent of Public Instruction) may have been here. We talked this all through. We presented what we thought good requirements ought to be. Dean Peterson and the people from the College of Education faculty spoke. And the people from the State Department would listen to them. So we got some changes made then which did

very much bolster our position.

The change that followed that Iowa City conference recognized people in speech correction as specialists who were different from classroom teachers and who did not have to meet the same requirements as classroom teachers but had their own requirements, in depth, in their specialty. Although students would still have to take a fair amount of coursework that would inform them about basic philosophy and history, operation of the public school system, et cetera, they did not have to meet the full certification requirements as teachers. At the same time they were required, however, to take a much more intensive program of work in the special field.

Darley and ISHA

In 1955 Darley was president of ISHA. He recalls *(2)* that he and his officers tried to make the Association's publication, *The Iowa Therapist,* a "more effective vehicle for communicating information about training programs and service programs." In some issues they developed a special section, with invited articles to cover some particular topic. One of these, for example, was about cleft palate.

Workshops

Summer workshops became a fairly routine part of the activities of the Iowa Program. These were concerned with a variety of subjects, often tied in with other projects in which there was a particular interest at the time. The workshop for the summer of 1953 is a case in point. Its subject was public school speech correction. Lectures were given by Johnson on stuttering; by Curtis and Sherman on voice and articulation disorders; by Spriestersbach and Nora Ames Ricci of the State Services for Crippled Children on cleft palate; by Darley and Dorothy Williams of the Hospital School on cerebral palsy; by Schubert, Reger, and Josephine Carr of the School for the Deaf on problems in hearing; by James Stroud of Education, Arthur Benton of Psychology (later of Psychology and Neurology), W. Grant Dahlstron, visiting professor in Psychology, and Jean Parker of the Children's Hospital on diagnosis and appraisal.

SSCC and the Hospital School

Johnson was president of the Iowa State Services for Crippled Children in 1953. Other faculty members were considerably involved in the work of that organization. The whole area of work with physically handicapped children was beginning to develop, with the establishment of the Hospital School for Severely Handicapped Children (now called the Hospital

School) by legislative action in 1947, and the subsequent interdisciplinary projects involving that institution and the Program. The School operated in a section of Westlawn from the fall of 1948 until January 1954 when its new (and present) building was ready for use.

ASHA

The Johnson period opened with Iowa trained Herbert Koepp-Baker as president of the American Speech and Hearing Association. Between then and the end of the period four others with Iowa Ph.D.s held that office: Delyte W. Morris in 1949, Johnson in 1950, Mack Steer in 1951, and Margaret Hall Powers in 1954. Johnson also doubled as chairman of the ASHA Midcentury White House Conference Committee during his presidential year.

During the period, five with Iowa Ph.D.s received Honors of the Association: Travis in 1947, Morris in 1949, Clarence Simon in 1950, Sara Stinchfield Hawk in 1953, and Fairbanks in 1955.

It is interesting to note that although the situation was eventually "remedied," Reger was *not* a member of ASHA. He wasn't eligible. The reason, he explains with some merriment, was that he had not taken the required courses. All he had done was teach them!

Other Iowa contributions and activities on the national scene in this period included Brown's election as ASHA vice-president while he was at Iowa, serving in 1948. He, Johnson, Fairbanks, and Curtis also served as councillors at various times during the period. Strother also served as a councillor soon after he left Iowa.

In 1948 Johnson completed six years as editor of the *Journal of Speech and Hearing Disorders* (called the *Journal of Speech Disorders* until 1947; he helped initiate the name change). His work in that office was recognized formally at the 1948 ASHA convention in a resolution which was printed in the March 1949 *Journal* (p. 2) and which carried this sentence: "His development of a scientific and scholarly journal has provided an essential voice for the field of speech and hearing; clinicians, teachers, and those engaged in research have been guided to improved description of their work, and to more effective expression of their ideas; through this dignified influence the Association has gained greatly in prestige." One of the great changes Johnson had made when he succeeded G. Oscar Russell, of Ohio State, the *Journal's* first editor, was to use material related to work being done in this country. Russell had printed European scholars almost exclusively.

Johnson's staff included four whose names had been closely associated with the Program in an earlier day: Hawk of Scripps College and Simon of Northwestern as associate editors; Ernest Henrikson of the University of

Colorado, later of Minnesota, as book review editor; Koepp-Baker, then on duty at the United States Naval hospital, Philadelphia, as war notes editor. Morris (Iowa Ph.D. 1936), then of Indiana State Teachers College, was Association business manager.

Fairbanks followed Johnson as editor of the *Journal*. On his staff Curtis served as an associate editor in the areas of speech science and statistical problems, and Brown in psychological problems and medical problems. Sherman was abstracts editor in 1955. (Fairbanks at this time was at the University of Illinois, in a small Iowa "colony": George Stoddard, president of the University, E. Thayer Curry and George Wischner, with Fairbanks in speech pathology and audiology.)

In 1950, the year of Johnson's presidency, the Association initiated its monograph series, supplements to the *Journal of Speech and Hearing Disorders*. The first four were issued during the Johnson period in 1950, 1952, 1953, and 1954. The fourth, "A Rationale for Articulation Disorders," was by Iowa-trained Robert Milisen of the University of Indiana and his students.

PUBLICATIONS

A strong publications program was supported during this period as in those preceding. Articles coming out of the work at Iowa were numerous, and were presented in a wide variety of scholarly journals as well as in selected segments of the popular press. Beyond this, faculty members contributed material, often chapters, to books produced by others, and five members of the faculty produced three books at Iowa. These three were: *Stuttering in Children and Adults (7)*, mentioned above; *Diagnostic Manual in Speech Correction (10)*, a text-workbook by Johnson, Darley, and Spriestersbach, published in 1952; and *Speech Handicapped School Children (9)*, a college-level textbook by Johnson, Brown, Curtis, and Keaster, plus Clarence Edney of the Speech Department, edited by Johnson, published in 1948. A second edition of the latter was being prepared at the end of the period and would appear in print in 1956.

TELEVISION AND RADIO

The Iowa Program reached many people by way of television and radio during the Johnson period. Programs included one called "New Hope for Stutterers," a part of the 1954-55 CBS television series, "The Search." Another was a presentation by the Iowa stuttering team on the NBC network from Chicago in 1950. Two programs on stuttering were telecast from WOI, Ames, in 1952 and 1954, for the Iowa State Medical Society.

Radio broadcasts were made from many stations over the country, often by Johnson. He was interviewed by Mary Margaret McBride in New York in 1951, 1953, and 1955.

MAY 1955

By 1955 the Program had reached a point of great vigor. Johnson mentioned this early that year in a lecture to students in Darley's course, introduction to clinical practice. Then he concluded by saying, "These remain our basic policies as we expand and move forward: On a firm and ever-renewing foundation of research and interdisciplinary teamwork we try to improve continuously our understandings, our professional training methods and standards, and our practical principles and procedures of prevention and remedial services. It is all right to know the answers only if you know what questions to ask in order to get better answers."

As early as February of 1955, some two months after he had had a heart attack, Johnson decided that in his remaining years he wanted to be relieved of administrative duties so that he could give himself more fully to the classroom and the clinic and the laboratory. Accordingly, he began to share with Curtis, his onetime student and his colleague since 1942, certain administrative duties. He did this increasingly in the months following so that in May, when he officially concluded his duties as administrator, and when Curtis officially assumed them, the changeover had already been accomplished.

THE WAY IT WAS

Not long ago in an interview Spriestersbach was asked about the climate in the Johnson period. Did he, for example, recall any experiences that had stayed with him. "Well, yes," he answered after a little thought, "these three in particular."

The first concerned a time of anxiety, when he and Oliver Bloodstein (Ph.D. 1948) took their final written examinations before the defense of their theses. "We were naturally apprehensive. And a couple of days later we met Johnson in the hall outside the speech clinic office. And he put his arm around my shoulder and said something like 'You did real well.' I don't remember his exact words. What I remember was that this fleeting act wasn't maudlin. It wasn't sentimental. It was momentary. He didn't make a big thing of it. Yet it was so warm. And so sincere. And I think a glimpse of the greatness of the man."

The second recollection was of a time of panic in the fall of 1948.

I had finished my work for the doctorate the end of May and about two weeks later was faced with the responsibility of teaching two courses in the summer session. The summer sessions are bad enough but I managed. Then came fall and I taught introduction to speech pathology as well as voice and articulation disorders and it became quite apparent to me that I was going to have to direct the research of a number of graduate students. Right after the war their number jumped very much, especially at the M.A. level. We had about 50 M.A. candidates at the time. The staff was much smaller than it is now and we hadn't gone to the nonthesis degree, so each graduate student had to have a thesis and somebody had to supervise it.

And I didn't have any questions to ask, questions to be investigated. I was panicked by this. And I remember going over to the D and L with Johnson for coffee and telling him my problem. He sipped his coffee a little bit and then he said, "You know, the thing you should do is take a topic and decide that you are going to know the most of anybody about that topic. If you'd do that, first thing you know you have more questions to be answered than you'll ever have time to answer. For example," he said, "take the /s/ sound. Consider the production of /s/ and all the problems in the articulation of this sound. Really study it. And you will have a whole program of research." Well, I never studied the /s/ sound but I never forgot what he said. I have cited it so many times in my teaching. It was wonderful advice to me. It gave me a point of view. And I think in many ways I followed his advice. When I got involved in the area of cleft palate I did this with velopharyngeal closure. I became pretty knowledgeable about this. And it was true that the more you learn, the more you know you don't know, and the first thing you know you are starting to throw out questions and students get interested and then you have a whole group doing research with you.

And I have gone back to that incident so many times in my lectures here and there, and I think I have always mentioned it in the introduction to research seminar, because it was so helpful to me. Mine was a terribly naive question that day really. But that answer was the right kind of advice at the right moment for me. I think that is the great secret of so much counseling and it was something that Johnson had such sensitivity to, such a true sense of when was the right time to do something or to say something.

The third recollection was not tied up with a particular incident, but had to do with the coloration, the very climate, of the Johnson period.

We were constantly reminded that there are no knowers and that this is a new field and the only way we can know about things is to study them and ask questions and do the research and all that. The emphasis was on ideas, not things. And this was always the way we operated in East Hall. So we really weren't bothered as I recall by the lack of therapy rooms and all that. What we were concerned about was knowing how to ask the questions, and understanding the basic, fundamental issues. These then we could adapt wherever we were and in whatever we were trying to do with the communication disorders. And when we would get involved in some facet of a problem, get terribly fascinated, completely immersed, it was Johnson who would bring things back into perspective for us. "Communication," he would say, "is the issue." I remember this happened many times. He never wanted us to lose sight of the broader view.

THE "IOWA MYSTIQUE"

William Tiffany, Iowa Ph.D. 1951, of the University of Washington, who was editor of the *Journal of Speech and Hearing Disorders* from 1962 to 1965, was also asked recently about his recollections of Iowa in the Johnson period. He *(21)* referred to what he called the "Iowa mystique" of the forties and fifties. This, it seemed to him, was compounded of many things, among them these eight, "probably in unequal parts":

Pride in the scholarly and research accomplishments of the present and past staff;

A sense of history—that it all started here and that the start itself grew out of a long line of deep and valid scholarship;

A sense of mission—that real human problems lay just outside our wall and that we could and would solve those problems;

The charismatic quality of Wendell Johnson's leadership;

A sense, as students, of being where the action was;

A sense of close identification between faculty and graduate students, of working in a common cause;

A sense that at Iowa our efforts were valued by others outside of our own department, together with the realization of our own debt to scholars in other disciplines; and

A twist of scholarly philosophy which made us feel that we were genuinely brought into a partnership in which we were tossing out the old didactic approaches to learning in favor of something both more valid and more human.

Then Tiffany adds, "Much lip service has been paid to this last, both before and since. I believe we really felt this as graduate students. Our morale was something I would like to recapture for my own students."

REFERENCES

1. James F. Curtis, taped conversations with author, Iowa City, June 24, 1968, November 22, 1968, January 31, 1969, January 24, 1972.

2. Frederic L. Darley, correspondence with author, January 30, 1969.

3. Wendell Johnson, correspondence with Ann M. Flowers, University of Virginia, May 1964 (information for dissertation).

4. Wendell Johnson, "Self-Reflexive Method of Clinical Counseling," undated (circa 1961) and unpublished manuscript, Johnson archives, University of Iowa Library.

5. Wendell Johnson, Sigma Alpha Eta faculty key address, Northwestern University, April 20, 1959, unpublished, Johnson archives, University of Iowa Library.

6. Wendell Johnson, "The Speech Correction Foundation," *Journal of Speech and Hearing Disorders, 13,* 1948, 49-50.

7. Wendell Johnson (Ed.), *Stuttering in Children and Adults* (Minneapolis: University of Minnesota Press, 1955).

8. Wendell Johnson and others, *The Onset of Stuttering* (Minneapolis: University of Minnesota Press, 1959).

9. Wendell Johnson, James Curtis, Spencer Brown, Clarence Edney, and Jacqueline Keaster, *Speech Handicapped School Children* (New York: Harper & Row, 1948, 1956, 1967; Johnson (Ed.), 1948, 1956; Johnson and Dorothy Moeller (Ed.), 1967).

10. Wendell Johnson, Frederic L. Darley, and D. C. Spriestersbach, *Diagnostic Manual in Speech Correction* (New York: Harper & Row, 1952).

11. Don Lewis and Dorothy Sherman, "Measuring the Severity of Stuttering," *Journal of Speech and Hearing Disorders, 16,* 1951, 320-326.

12. Dean Lierle, taped interview with author, Iowa City, September 24, 1969.

13. Michael Marge, "State Speech and Hearing Associations," *Asha, 9,* September 1967, 343-7.

14. Milton Metfessel, "Carl Emil Seashore, 1866-1949," *Science, 111,* 1950, 713-17.

15. Scott Reger, taped conversation with author, Iowa City, April 3, 1968.

16. Earl D. Schubert, "Research Study of the Psycho-Acoustic Effects of Human and Artificial Sidetone," The University of Iowa, Army, Project 3-99-12-022, Contract DA36-039, sc42562, *Final Report,* 1954 (Atkinson series).

17. Mrs. Earl D. Schubert, correspondence with author, May 24, 1969.

18. Jeanne Kellenberger Smith, conversation and correspondence with author, Iowa City, October and November 1971, and March 1972.

19. D. C. Spriestersbach, taped conversation with author, Iowa City, January 24, 1969.

20. Charles Strother, taped conversation with author, Chicago, March 1, 1968.

21. William Tiffany, correspondence with author, March 20, 1968.

22. Joseph Tiffin, "Carl Emil Seashore, 1866-1949," *Psychological Review, 57,* 1950, 1-2.

23. Lee Edward Travis, taped conversation with author, Los Angeles, February 28, 1968.

24. Lee Edward Travis (Ed.), *Handbook of Speech Pathology* (New York: Appleton-Century-Crofts, 1957).

NOTES

[1] Memos and documents not identified in another way are from the University archives in the University Library.

[2] Hancher had assumed the presidency in 1940, succeeding Eugene Gilmore, who had served from 1934 to 1940. Gilmore, in turn, had succeeded Walter A. Jessup, known as a builder of the University and a supporter and friend of the Program. Jessup was president from 1916 to 1934. Chester A. Phillips, dean of the College of Commerce (now Business Administration), was acting president for about three months between the Gilmore and Hancher administrations.

[3] Although it is beyond the time span covered in the present writing, the October 1970 semicentennial celebration of the Psychopathic Hospital's founding stands as a third "reunion." Travis was a featured speaker and others of the Travis period took part in the event which was planned by Dr. Paul Huston and his colleagues.

[4] Records cited in this section, and in the section entitled "Speech Correction in State Institutions," are from the files of the Department of Speech Pathology and Audiology unless another source is indicated.

8

THE CURTIS PERIOD: 1955-1968

When James F. Curtis became principal administrative officer of the Program, that is, Chairman of the Council on Speech Pathology and Audiology, in the spring of 1955, he was entering on a term of service that would be longer than that of any of his predecessors—thirteen years, compared with eleven for Lee Travis and eight each for Charles Strother and Wendell Johnson. By the end of his term in September 1968, when he chose to leave administration in favor of full-time teaching and research, Curtis and his colleagues had: seen the creation of the Department of Speech Pathology and Audiology at Iowa; taken a leadership role nationally in development of the discipline and of professional standards within the discipline; been particularly active in working for federal support of training and research in speech pathology and audiology and related fields; been involved in major projects made possible by increasing grant support; reorganized the Iowa clinical services program; expanded and revised curricula; and had moved into the Wendell Johnson Speech and Hearing Center, a new building designed and equipped for the Department, and named to memorialize the work Johnson had done for the enterprise.

The Curtis leadership within the Department was seen particularly in the curriculum changes which shifted the major part of professional training to the graduate level and provided broadened basic training, strong in speech and hearing science, at the undergraduate level. Curtis had worked in speech science since his days as a doctoral candidate, following in the line of Dean Carl E. Seashore, Travis, Milton Metfessel, Joseph Tiffin, Grant Fairbanks, and Gladys Lynch. By 1960 he could report[1] to Dean Dewey B. Stuit of the College of Liberal Arts that, "although the Department is not formally organized into divisions, both staff and courses can be grouped into three major categories: speech pathology, audiology, and speech and hearing science." By the end of the period, in addition to the strengthened undergraduate offerings, a full graduate program had been developed in speech and hearing science, joining those established earlier in speech pathology and in audiology.

FACULTY DURING THE CURTIS PERIOD (1955-1968)

When Curtis became chairman of the Council on Speech Pathology and Audiology his faculty numbered seven: himself, Johnson, Spriestersbach, Darley, Sherman, Schubert, and Parker. By 1968, the closing year of the Curtis period (and of the present writing), the faculty included Curtis, Spriestersbach, and Sherman from the original seven. According to the listing in University catalogue No. 1968, the Department Staff list carried twenty-six names, and the Affiliated Staff list carried five more. During the time span of the Curtis period there were shifts of emphasis, realignments, and general growth, all intimately related to the work of earlier years. Something of the shape of the development can be told in terms of the work of the seven on that beginning faculty.

Speech Science. The speech science area developed under the direction of Curtis, who also continued to head the Phonetics and Speech Laboratory in the Department of Speech. When the curriculum in the Department of Speech Pathology and Audiology was revised later in his administration to expand fundamental offerings at the undergraduate level, Kenneth Moll (Iowa Ph.D. 1960) taught the phonetics course and fundamentals of speech science. Moll had been appointed to the faculty in 1959, serving first on the Spriestersbach cleft palate project (see below).

GS, Counseling, and Stuttering. Johnson carried on in general semantics, symbolic processes, clinical counseling, and stuttering. Dean Williams (Iowa Ph.D. 1952) returned to Iowa from Indiana University to join the Department faculty in 1957 and to assume responsibility for the work in stuttering. Johnson then moved more and more into the study of communication in relation to human problems. Williams' responsibilities developed in such a way that he was in charge of most of the clinical work in the Department, in addition to his own growing program of teaching and research in the area of stuttering, and all of this complicated by the fact that the clinical caseload was increasing. Clinical associates named in these years included Bette Spriestersbach (Iowa M.A. 1945) in 1963; Linda Smith Jordan (Iowa M.A. 1964) and Aaron Favors (Iowa Ph.D. 1969) in 1964; Marie Emge (Iowa M.A. 1958) in 1965; Elaine Dripps (Boston M.Ed. 1958) and Judith Milisen Knabe (Wisconsin M.S. 1964) in 1967.

Cleft Palate. D. C. Spriestersbach was involved primarily with work in the area of problems associated with cleft palate. At the beginning of the period he entered on the development of the major and ongoing project which since 1955, and with significant grant support, has brought the Department of Speech Pathology and Audiology into a collaborative relationship with the Department of Otolaryngology and Maxillofacial Surgery in the investigation of sociopsychological and anatomical-physiological aspects of cleft palate. When Hughlett Morris (Iowa Ph.D. 1961) joined the faculty in 1960, he began his duties in the clinical part of Spriestersbach's project. At that time Moll's work centered in the cinematography laboratory there. As Spriestersbach became more involved with responsibilities at the national level—with the National Institutes of Health and the American Speech and Hearing Association—Morris took over some of his teaching in cleft palate. And when Spriestersbach became dean of the Graduate College in 1965, Morris took over his role in the project. Duane Van Demark (Iowa Ph.D. 1962), appointed to the faculty in 1965, assumed the clinical duties Morris had carried.

At the beginning of the period, Spriestersbach also taught the introductory course in speech pathology and audiology, as he had before, and in that devised a team-teaching approach with various faculty members coming in to lecture. Johnson was in charge of the course for a time; so was Williams; so also was James Neelley (Iowa Ph.D. 1960), who served on the staff on a temporary basis. Throughout the Curtis period, Spriestersbach continued to teach a seminar in introduction to research methods.

Organic Disorders, Diagnosis and Appraisal. Darley continued, as in the Johnson period, in the area of organic speech disorders other than cleft palate, in neuropathologies of speech, and in diagnosis and appraisal. The latter was renamed introduction to clinical procedures and, after Darley's resignation in 1960, to join the staff of the Mayo Clinic, was taught by Evan Jordan (Iowa Ph.D. 1961), who joined the faculty in 1960.

The part of Darley's work that was concerned with organic speech problems became the responsibility of James Hardy (Iowa Ph.D. 1961), who had been supervisor of speech and hearing services in the Hospital School and who for a while after his appointment to the Department faculty in 1960 divided his time between the Department and administration of speech and hearing services in the Hospital School. It was then that he began his major sponsored research program in respiratory physiology, particularly in the area of problems of children with cerebral palsy. He developed his laboratory in the Hospital School and then, when the new Speech and Hearing Center opened, moved it there.

Public School Work, Research, Voice and Articulation. Sherman, from the beginning of the Curtis period, continued with her work in public school speech correction methods, research design, and voice and articulation disorders. In the period of her editorship of the *Journal of Speech and Hearing Research,* 1958-1963, the latter was taught by Jordan for a short time, also by Richard McDermott (Iowa Ph.D. 1962), then later was shared by her and Morris. The public school work was reorganized in the general reorganization of clinical services in 1965. About that same time Sherman assumed responsibility for the honors program within the Department.

Audiology (the initial period). The situation in audiology was fluid for several years, perhaps reflecting the facts that the science, as such, was new, and that these were years of adjustment for the discipline itself. This beginning period may be said to have extended from 1955 to 1963. Schubert, who had laid the foundation for the work in the Department, resigned in 1955. By then there was at least the beginning of definition in three areas: basic audition, that is, basic work in psychoacoustics; clinical activities in audition including testing; and rehabilitative work with individuals with hearing problems.

Reger's coursework in Otolaryngology and Lewis's in Psychology had been in the area of psychoacoustics, as had Schubert's, and for a short time after Schubert left, Parker taught in this area even though his interests centered in the clinical. Juergen Tonndorf (Kiel M.D. 1938) of Otolaryngology taught coursework in electrophysiology in audition.

Curtis and his colleagues decided to bring in a person whose specific training was in sensory psychology with an emphasis in audition. This person was Arnold Small (Wisconsin Ph.D. 1954), who was appointed to the faculty in 1957.

The acoustics course, which had begun with the Stewart tradition in physics in the Travis days, had been phased out for all practical purposes after several years in which it had been taught by graduate students in physics as a joint offering of Music and Speech Pathology and Audiology. Richard Voots (Iowa Ph.D. 1955) in 1961 was engaged to teach this.

At the beginning of the Curtis period, the plan had been that Parker would expand the clinical work in audition. He decided, however, to accept a position at Montana, and left Iowa in 1956. James Shapley (Iowa Ph.D. 1954), who had been appointed to the faculty in 1955, continued the clinical activities. When he resigned in 1959, the responsibilities passed to William Prather (Iowa Ph.D. 1960), who was named to the faculty that year. Prather resigned in 1962 and was succeeded by Malcolm Hast (Ohio State Ph.D. 1961).

Rehabilitative work in audiology had been primarily the responsibility of Keaster, who had resigned in 1953. The program was expanding rapidly, and the Keaster duties in the Department of Otolaryngology were assumed by Jeanne K. Smith (Iowa M.A. 1937) and in the Department of Speech Pathology and Audiology by Parker, then, in turn, by Shapley and Hast.

Audiology (after 1963). Early in the sixties the Department staff developed a plan for the expansion of work in audiology. The feeling was that this should include five areas: basic psychoacoustics, which was Small's area; clinical audiology, which would include supervision of the clinical program and teaching in coursework; research which would combine psychoacoustics research with practical problems of testing persons with hearing problems and which, then, would be directed toward developing procedures in testing; rehabilitative audiology, which would include auditory training, hearing conservation as such, language problems of persons with hearing loss; and neurophysiological research.

Psychoacoustics was being taken care of by Small, of course, but the implementation of the rest of the plan began in 1963 with the appointment of Jay Melrose (Illinois Ph.D. 1954) and Cletus Fisher (Ohio State Ph.D. 1963), and continued the next year with the appointment of David Lilly (Pittsburgh Ph.D. 1961). Responsibilities of Melrose were in clinical audiology; those of Fisher, in rehabilitative audiology; those of Lilly, in research on testing procedures. (Development of the fifth area, neurophysiological research, began after the end of the Curtis period with the appointment of Joel Wernick [Stanford Ph.D. 1967].) Fisher succeeded Hast, whose training was in biophysics, and who then shifted back to that area after a brief time in audiology. He became a full-time member of the staff in Otolaryngology, doing research on laryngeal function.

The 1965 reorganization of the Speech Clinic and of clinical services, which had become the responsibility of Williams, meant that Melrose, who had a joint appointment in Otolaryngology and Speech Pathology and Audiology, moved entirely into the latter when he became director of clinical services of the Department of Speech Pathology and Audiology. He was succeeded in Otolaryngology by Charles Anderson (Pittsburgh Ph.D. 1962), who began his work at Iowa in 1966. (Melrose began his joint appointment in 1963 as director of the audiology section in Otolaryngology. He became head of speech pathology and audiology in Otolaryngology in 1964, and carried that duty and also the duty of director of Clinical Services in Speech Pathology and Audiology the following year. In 1966 he was able to move entirely into the latter.)

Another Laboratory. An addition to the resources on which the Department drew during the Curtis period was the mobile field clinic program of the State Services for Crippled Children. Carl Betts (Iowa Ph.D. 1963), consultant in speech and hearing for the SSCC, officially became a member of the Department staff the year of his degree, although he had been making contributions to the Department before then, through the mobile clinic program. As his program expanded, students from the Department were given the opportunity of laboratory experience in testing and evaluating working with the mobile-clinic staff. Betts' teaching in the Department was in the area of language development, with emphasis on that development in mentally retarded children. He continued as head consultant for SSCC in speech and language problems, and took over Hardy's responsibilities as supervisor of speech and hearing services in the Hospital School.

Another Area. In 1965, Arthur Compton (Ohio State Ph.D. 1965) was named to the faculty to develop work in psycholinguistics, which was a new area for the curriculum. His basic work was in speech acquisition processes of young children, later to be expanded to include relearning of language in adults, as in cases of brain damage.

In Summary. One kind of summary of the growth in Department resources during the Curtis period was presented in the literature prepared for the dedication of the new Speech and Hearing Center. It was this alphabetical listing of the areas in which the Department offered work: acoustics; anatomy and physiology of speech and auditory processes; articulation disorders; audiometry; aural rehabilitation; cleft palate; clinical procedures; development of speech and language; hearing science; neural processes and neuropathologies of speech and language; pathologies of audition; phonetics; psychoacoustics; psycholinguistics; speech science; stuttering; and voice disorders.

INTERDISCIPLINARY ACTIVITY

The Program's tradition of interdisciplinary activity continued to be honored by Curtis as it had been by Travis, Strother, and Johnson before him. A 1962 University News and Information Service release, written by Johnson and Williams, included this paragraph about it:

> In pioneering the new profession, Dean Seashore and his associates laid down a basic principle that still governs the SUI Speech Pathology and Audiology Program—the principle of cutting across departmental and college lines in order to bring to bear on the problems to be solved all of the resources of the University. This principle has made the SUI program the most productive in the world. Iowa leads all other universities in the number of Ph.D. degrees granted in speech pathology and audiology; in the number of its graduates who are directors of clinics, laboratories, and training programs; in the number of Fellows and present and past officers of the American Speech and Hearing Association; in the amount of research and the number of research publications in speech and hearing.

MABIE, STEWART, LYNCH

The interdisciplinary activity, and indeed the total undertaking, may be said to have lost three of its staunchest supporters when, early in the period and within a span of only fourteen months, three longtime friends of the Program died: Edward C. Mabie, virtual head of the enterprise for two decades, February 9, 1956; George Stewart, head of the Physics Department who had made his classrooms and laboratories available to the Program for work in acoustics, August 16, 1956; and Gladys Lynch, a pioneer in speech science who had studied with Travis and had taught with

Fairbanks and Curtis, April 16, 1957.

Mabie. Although Mabie had come into the Program by the accident of Glenn Merry's leave of absence, and although his training was in the theater, he not only accommodated to the new Seashore-Travis scientific approach to speech, but also became one of its important and effective supporters. He had then proceeded to take on a leadership role in the Program, a role more or less thrust on him by circumstance. While the formation of the Council on Speech Pathology and Audiology in 1951 had taken care of some of the administrative difficulties related to the Program, he appears to have continued an active search for a better solution. In a memorandum of May 1952, for example, he suggests to his faculty five "possible ways of reorganizing" the Department of Speech, in all five recognizing speech pathology and audiology as a major unit.

By 1956 his budget carried almost the total Program and his Department was in large measure its home. Many developmental changes were his work. A case in point is his presentation to the University administration which resulted in space and equipment for Curtis's speech and phonetics laboratory, which in turn led to Curtis's decision to remain at Iowa rather than to accept an offer from another institution.

Bryng Bryngelson, who earned his M.S. at Iowa in 1926 and his Ph.D. in 1931, remembers *(1)* warmly the "good spirit of E. C. Mabie" in bringing Charles Woolbert to the Iowa faculty in 1926 at a salary of "$500 more than Mr. Mabie was getting," and of offering any help he could give in finding Bryngelson a position after the M.S., when Bryngelson was not in a position to go on with graduate work.

Those who worked with Mabie recall his enthusiasm for new ideas, and his encouragement in putting them to the test. Spriestersbach *(10)* has many memories of this. The May 1952 memorandum mentioned above also illustrates the point. After listing his five plans, Mabie added as a sixth: "You make a plan and bring it to the meeting."

Strother *(11)* describes him as "unpredictable, stimulating, and complex." The faculty memorial statement at the time of his death cites his "constant drive to attain the high ideals which he set for himself and his associates, both students and faculty." The statement then continues, " . . . perhaps Professor Mabie's life is best characterized by the sentence: he made big plans. He was one of those who started the interdisciplinary work in speech science and speech pathology on this campus and in the nation, and helped it grow locally to its eminent position."

Stewart. For Stewart, creativity was one of the highest ideals of intellectual activity. His discussions of this subject in the classroom, later rather formally with groups in his home, became widely known on the campus. Perhaps it was this personal orientation that led him to support so strongly the pioneering venture represented by the Program.

Like Mabie, he was known internationally. His contribution to the Program is seen as reflecting both this professional excellence in the field of acoustics and his unusual enthusiasm for the creative process. In other words, along with subject matter he contributed a point of view, an orientation to creative scholarship.

Lynch. After starting out as an English major, Lynch found herself increasingly fascinated by the anatomy and function of the speech mechanism. So it was that she came into the Program for her doctoral work with Travis, earning her Ph.D. in 1932. She first taught at Winona State Teachers College and it was there she had as a student one D. C. Spriestersbach, whom she interested in coming to Iowa. She returned to the Iowa campus to join the faculty of the Speech Department in 1943, from then on teaching in its speech science area.

She is said to have demanded much of her classes, and she gave much in return. It was only after her death that her colleagues and students were to discover how very much she gave, how many she had helped, how many kindnesses she had managed that only she and the recipient knew about. Spriestersbach, for example, she sponsored for a scholarship, then loaned support money "on which to live; all at her initiative—not at my request," he adds *(10).*

COUNCIL TO DEPARTMENT

In the official record there is a statement that the Department of Speech Pathology and Audiology was established in 1956, a perfectly adequate statement for the purpose there, but not very informative for those interested in knowing just how such an historic event took place. In answer to a question about this, Curtis *(2)* began by explaining that the situation was probably "not typical" because over a period of years the Program had become increasingly autonomous until by this time it was almost completely so.

He went on to say,

> We dealt with the Graduate College in a very direct fashion, not going through any intermediate administrative level. We dealt with the Registrar's office on matters of admission. We made our own decisions about curriculum. So to all practical purposes we were a department, in everything but name almost. We had a budget page that came to us from Mabie's office, and so on.
>
> The feeling had been developing among all of the faculty then involved that it was but a matter of time and probably a relatively short time before we should actually be granted departmental status and before we would take action to bring this about.
>
> But I think we all shared a feeling that Mabie, over the years, had

had a tremendous interest in the development of the Program in Speech Pathology and Audiology and speech science and that he had encouraged that development to the best of his ability and had done a great deal to help it grow and develop. And we did not want to seem to him to be ungrateful for all of this and unappreciative of this. We did not want him to feel there was anything personal in such action. And so during his tenure I think there was some reluctance to proceed on this.

After his death, the issue had to be faced immediately. There were reasons to think of us, on some sort of administrative chart, as a division of the Department of Speech and Dramatic Art although Johnson had always characterized us as a free-floating program with roots in many areas and departments and not contained wholly within any one. And this was the way we thought of ourselves. Mabie had understood this. But with another administrator this might not be so. Besides we felt that we had achieved a stature worthy of recognition as a department and this seemed the time to do it. So we raised the issue at the time discussions began in the naming of a successor to Mabie.

The matter was not settled without a considerable amount of discussion and, sometimes, rather heated controversy. There were, of course, many points of view to be considered for this was a complex matter for all concerned. There were several meetings in which other members of the Department of Speech and Dramatic Art were involved and we were involved. Basically we presented the case for a department and the others, for the most part, argued against it, and Dean Stuit was caught in between. We became very insistent. And although I am sure he would like to have had a unanimous directive from all concerned, that did not develop. After much consideration he made the decision in our favor, transmitting through channels his own favorable recommendation along with our request and recommendation.

The recommendations in turn were acted upon favorably by the administration. The Department of Speech Pathology and Audiology was established July 1 of that year [1956].

BEYOND THE CAMPUS

Curtis and his colleagues became very active very early in his administration working for legislation which would provide federal support for training and research in speech pathology and audiology and related fields. Their accomplishments, of course, benefited programs across the nation as well as at Iowa.

At the public hearings for the initial legislation, for example, held in Chicago in May 1960, Curtis presented (2) the case for speech pathology and audiology, emphasizing to United States Representative Carl Elliott's

Subcommittee on Special Education of the House Committee on Education and Labor that this discipline was not a part of special education, as others were suggesting. It contributed to special education, he pointed out, but emphasized that there was much more to speech pathology and audiology and to education of the deaf than was contained in departments of special education in colleges and universities, or in special education administrative units in the schools. Interestingly enough, speech and hearing were the first of the various areas sometimes called special education to have any federal grant support.

Johnson had a very large impact on the whole legislative program, Curtis feels.

> He was well acquainted with people in key positions in several agencies in the Washington scene. He was a very good friend of Richard Masland of NINDS—it was then NINDB[2]—and he was well acquainted with Mary Switzer in the Office of Vocational Rehabilitation. He was also acquainted with people in the Office of Education.
>
> He had an off-campus assignment for much of the academic year of 1957-58 to serve as consultant to the Office of Education and to NINDB. And he spent a good deal of time in Vocational Rehabilitation. And I am sure that he had a great deal to do with the way in which the direction of the thinking that led to the legislation went, that is, to the extent that the legislation was influenced by the people in those offices and I think it was influenced very greatly.

As the federally supported programs developed in the various agencies, several people from the Iowa faculty were selected to fill positions in which they participated in reviewing research grant and training grant proposals. Spriestersbach was very active with the National Institute of Dental Research, later becoming chairman of their training grants committee. He served, as well, a full term on the speech and hearing training panel of the Office of Education and a three-year term on the training committee of both NINDB and NIDR. Dean Williams was active on review panels for the Office of Education and for the Vocational Rehabilitation Administration. Curtis was involved primarily with NINDB. He and Dr. Lierle and Earl Schubert, then no longer at Iowa, served on the original communicative sciences study section of NINDB. Dr. Brian McCabe, Dr. Lierle's successor in Otolaryngology and Maxillofacial Surgery, became a member later. So did Harry Hollein (Iowa Ph.D. 1955) and Paul Jensen (Iowa Ph.D. 1962). (There are seventeen members on this section, from a variety of disciplines. Curtis became a member of the section for the second time, again for a three-year term, later in the sixties; he became chairman in 1972.)

Beginning about 1965, Curtis served on a special subcommittee of the Council of NINDS to develop a report on human communication and its disorders, this report to be used by the Council as an advisory document in its decision-making process in matters concerned with training and research support. Curtis, Stanley Ainsworth (Iowa Ph.D. 1949), and Dr. Joseph Ogura of St. Louis formed a subcommittee of the committee to develop the section of the report on speech disorders as such. (The report was completed in 1969.)

ALSO ON THE NATIONAL SCENE

Other evidences of Iowa leadership beyond the campus were many. These take their place in the chronology of events in following pages, but, as a sampling, here are four:

Curtis was president of the American Speech and Hearing Association in 1962. Spriestersbach was president of the American Speech and Hearing Association in 1965 and president, also, of the American Cleft Palate Association in 1961-62. Frederic L. Darley was president of the Iowa Speech and Hearing Association in 1955, James C. Hardy in 1962, and Evan Jordan in 1965. Other faculty members assumed major committee responsibilities in all of these organizations. Carl Betts (Iowa Ph.D. 1963) and Dale Bingham (Iowa M.A. 1951) represented ISHA at the first meeting of the ASHA House of Delegates, before the Los Angeles convention of 1960. Other faculty people who have been representatives to the House are Jordan and Hughlett Morris. The Iowa Association was second in the nation, following Kentucky, to be accepted by the ASHA as a member of the ASHA House of Delegates. That action came in 1959.

In 1955 Dr. Lierle was instrumental in creating the Committee on the Conservation of Hearing for the State of Iowa, which the Department of Speech Pathology and Audiology has been involved in ever since. Members are representatives of those two departments, the State Department of Health, the Section on Otology of the Iowa State Medical Society, and the Division of Special Education of the State Department of Public Instruction. Sponsorship of the committee was assumed by the State Department of Health in 1957. Iowa people who have served on the Committee from 1955 through 1968, according to records made available by Jeanne K. Smith *(9)* are: *otolaryngology,* Dr. Lierle, Dr. C. M. Kos, Dr. McCabe, and Jeanne K. Smith, hearing consultant; *audiology,* Charles Parker, James Shapley, William Prather, Jay Melrose, Charles Anderson, and Malcolm Hast; *speech and hearing,* Curtis, Kenneth Moll, and Cletus Fisher.

One Thursday in August 1960 was to Johnson "an historic day," as he put it in a letter to a friend soon after.[3] He explained, "For nearly twenty years I have been *trying to get Speech Pathology recognized officially by the United States Civil Service Commission* as a profession in its own right and last Thursday we won. . . .We spent over three hours at the USCSC and it was about as gruelling a test as I have ever had in trying to present a case for something I believed in. What we accomplished was recognition by the USCSC of Speech Pathology as an independent profession."

The Speech Correction Fund, which traced its lineage back to Johnson's Demosthenes Club on the Iowa campus in the thirties, became the *American Speech and Hearing Foundation* as a result of ASHA action in 1956. The corporate structure adopted then is outlined in Article XV of the by-laws of the Association. Johnson, a founder of the Fund in 1945 and Chairman of the ASHA Fund committee from 1948, became Chairman of the Foundation at the time of its establishment, and held that position until shortly before his death in 1965.

In the early days of the Foundation, Johnson began to assign to it the royalties of his "Open Letter to the Mother of a 'Stuttering' Child" (*4*, pp. 543-554), a relatively small document he began writing in 1941 and revised over and over again, polishing, simplifying, often working at the rewriting on trains and in air terminals. Tens of thousands of copies of the Letter have been distributed, and it has been reprinted in other publications, including a Japanese speech text of which one author was Sumiko Sasanuma (Iowa Ph.D. 1968) who had studied with Johnson, among others.

In a brief historical sketch about the Foundation, Johnson (*3*) in 1960 listed among the scholarship winners of the previous year three men who later joined the Iowa faculty: David Lilly, then at the University of Pittsburgh, Evan Jordan, and Duane Van Demark, graduate students at Iowa.

THE GENERAL SITUATION

The Curtis period came at a time of remarkable growth and development in speech pathology and audiology as an academic discipline. One way to "see" this growth is to look at the membership totals of the American Speech and Hearing Association at landmark years in the Iowa history. From the first year of the Association in 1926 on through to the end of the Travis period in 1938, the membership grew from about 100 to 200. By 1947, the end of the Strother period, it was nearing 900. By 1951, the year the Iowa Council was established, it was 1,859. By 1955, the end of the Johnson period, it was 3,161. In 1956, when the Iowa Council became the Iowa Department, it stood at 3,974. It had passed the 10,000 mark by 1963 and by 1968, the end of the Curtis period, it was 13,000.

There was also a rapid increase in the number of institutions providing programs of study in this field. Prior to World War II the number of universities offering graduate study, especially at the doctoral level, was very limited. In the Big Ten only Iowa, Michigan, Northwestern, and

Wisconsin then offered recognized doctoral programs. In the remainder of the country there were four more: Columbia, Pennsylvania State University, Louisiana State University, and the University of Southern California. A few others were offering M.A. level programs. By 1957-58, there were 151 institutions offering bachelor's degrees, ninety offering master's degrees, and twenty-two offering doctor's degrees. In 1960-61 these numbers had increased to 183, 113, and 30, respectively.

DEPARTMENT REPORTS

When the Program became a Department it entered a system of departmental procedures, one of which involved department reports. Curtis, as chief administrative officer, wrote these reports at the specified times and submitted them, as required, to Dean Stuit. As a result, and for the first time since the Iowa Program began, an official and continuing record was thus being maintained, detailing the projects, progress, and problems of Speech Pathology and Audiology at Iowa. Records before this time were, like the Program itself, a part of something else and so were made up of fragments imbedded and all but lost in other records.

Curtis' 1960 Department Report may be considered something of a bench mark for developments of the period. By that year the work had reached such a point of definition that the activities described in that Report became major considerations from then on. They included, in the order in which they appear in the Report: the relationship of degree programs and career opportunities, the growing size and complexity of the service program and the need for an organizational change to cope with that growth, the curriculum challenges in the areas of clinical audiology and of speech and hearing science, the problems of adquate housing, and the range of research then in progress.

1960

In 1960 the Department was offering programs leading to the B.A., M.A., and Ph.D. degrees. According to that year's Report, persons at the B.A. level

> are either preparing for immediate vocational placement as speech correctionists in elementary and secondary schools or are preparing for specialized graduate training. Those for whom the M.A. is the terminal goal are preparing for positions in schools or special education programs calling for advanced training or are preparing for clinical service positions in hospitals, speech and hearing centers, rehabilitation centers, special schools for handicapped children, etc.
>
> Candidates for the Ph.D. degree are primarily preparing for

teaching and research positions in colleges and universities although many of these positions require a high degree of clinical competence also. In recent years a definite trend has developed toward full-time clinical positions demanding Ph.D. level training and it is expected that this trend will be intensified in the future. There has also been some demand in industrial and government laboratories for persons to carry on full-time research activity in speech and hearing science, especially related to communications engineering, and a beginning has been made toward providing degree programs for persons who wish to prepare for such careers.

Service Program. Because of the clinical competence required of many graduates, the

Department is necessarily engaged in an extensive service program in order to provide the clinical experiences required for competent preparation of such graduates. In addition to the services offered quite directly by the Department, which include the University Speech Clinic, the Outpatient Speech Clinic, and the Summer Residential Speech Clinic, this service program embraces speech and hearing services offered through the Department of Otolaryngology and Maxillofacial Surgery and the Department of Pediatrics of University Hospitals together with services provided by a number of agencies affiliated more or less closely with University Hospitals, such as the Hospital School for Severely Handicapped Children, the Child Development Clinic, State Services from Crippled Children, and the Iowa City Veterans Hospital. The expansion and development of these hospital affiliated services in speech pathology and audiology has been particularly significant and rapid in recent years. Coordination and supervision of this expanding service program has made increasing demands on staff time. The time is rapidly approaching when a general review of these services, looking toward a more efficient and effective organization of them, will be urgently needed.

(Later in the Report, Curtis points to the need, "felt for some years," to strengthen the clinical training program in the direction of increasing the staff by adding full-time professionally trained personnel with extensive clinical experience to supervise all practicum experience of students. The supervision at that time was being handled by members of the faculty, in addition to their regular teaching and research, and by graduate students.)

Courses. The 1960 Report continues that at that time the Department

offers an excellent program in speech pathology. Its teaching program in clinical audiology must be strengthened. The problems here include the facs that as a more or less separate specialized field it is relatively new; development of staff and program has been retarded by losses of key personnel; and, finally, integration of the

Department's program with that of the Department of Otolaryngology and Maxillofacial Surgery is required. This integration has now been accomplished. The necessary structure of courses, seminars, practicums, etc., has been planned. What remains to be done is to implement this planning by strengthening the staff in this area.

Dr. Lierle, commenting recently *(6)* on the cooperation of the Iowa Program and the Iowa Department of Speech Pathology and Audiology with his own Department of Otolaryngology and Maxillofacial Surgery, mentioned both Johnson's and Curtis's "interest in our work. They were very cooperative. We owe them a great deal." He spoke too of the "pleasant relationships" between the two departments and the contributions of these men to that. "And we don't want to forget Dr. Spriestersbach," he continued. "He was exceedingly helpful. He was the director of speech in our cleft lip and cleft palate clinic and obtained large grants from the National Institute of Health. He did an outstanding job while he was here. He was very cooperative, a tower of strength in this Department." And Morris, who succeeded Spriestersbach there, "has continued to do very good work."

The 1960 Department Report, after mention of work with the Department of Otolaryngology and Maxillofacial Surgery, continues with the statement that, "a second area which needs strengthening is that of speech and hearing science." The Report goes on:

Post World War II developments have seen a remarkable growth in research interest in this area by government and industrial laboratories. Up to the present time the teaching in this area of the Department has been mainly supportive in the sense of providing the necessary scientific background for students whose programs were primarily directed toward clinical interests in speech pathology and audiology. Opportunity of a limited sort has been provided for advanced courses and seminars and it has always been possible to carry out thesis research in nonclinical, scientific investigation of speech and hearing phenomena. A beginning [in strengthening the work in this direction] has been made in that a grant to support an expansion of graduate education in hearing science under Title IV of the National Defense Act has been approved.

Space Problems. Previous analyses

from this Department have emphasized that our present space is both inadequate and scattered so that operations can not be efficiently organized. This situation has continually become more critical. A comprehensive analysis of space needs requires decisions concerning the future organization of the service program in relation to University Hospitals and related facilities. Tentatively the recommendation would be to build a Speech and Hearing Center to provide facilities for a service and research program in conjunction with University Hospitals. Estimated cost would be $750,000. Of this approximately 60% would be available from federal grants. Needs from state funds would be the necessary matching funds, estimated at $300,000. [Both of the estimates proved low. See Contract Letting, 1965.]

The space problem "has been intensified by the various federal grant programs which have accrued in the past several years. We now have four substantial federal grants for research and two training grant programs." The latter were from the Office of Vocational Rehabilitation, wholly supporting the work of one faculty member, and from the Children's Bureau, partially supporting the work of two faculty members and ten graduate assistants.

Research. The major portion of staff research in stuttering was being conducted with support of the OVR grant, with Johnson as project director and Williams as associate director. "The purpose is to investigate and improve the effectiveness of clinical procedures with stutterers."

Cleft palate research was directed by Spriestersbach, supported by two grants from the National Institutes of Health. "The main direction of the Spriestersbach program," the Report continues,

is evaluation of diagnostic procedures and improvement of diagnostic methods. One aspect is investigation of physiological dynamics of the velopharyngeal valving mechanism by cineradiographic procedures, equipment for which has been bought be grant funds. [One of four major cleft-palate research centers in the United States was established in Otolaryngology with the purchase of this and related equipment.] A corollary aspect of this work, made possible by the laboratory equipment, is fundamental investigation of the physiology of speech articulation and correlation of such physiological data with acoustic data on speech articulation.

Through cooperative arrangements with the Hospital School a program of investigation of speech breathing is underway. Those involved principally are Curtis and Hardy. The work is concerned with investigating fundamental relationships of pulmonary function to speech, including basic data relating to normal speech and to speech in children with cerebral palsy. A substantial grant for continued support of this work has just been awarded by NIH to the Hospital School.

Research on hearing is proceeding under a grant from the National Science Foundation, directed by Small. This is basic research in psychoacoustics, specifically the pitch response to certain special types of acoustic pulse stimuli.

Other staff research includes that of Darley in cooperation with

Mildred Templin of Minnesota. He has just completed preparation for publication [*12*] of a diagnostic test for articulation skill in young children which is based on the best available normative data in this area. This is part of Darley's long-time interest in the development of language functions in children.

Research on psychological scaling procedures in the evaluation of speech behavior has been carried on by Sherman as for many years past. Her most recent interest has been in the method of direct magnitude estimation.

AN AWARD-WINNING EXHIBIT, 1961

In 1961 Hardy, Spriestersbach, Moll, and Morris won first award for their scientifiic exhibit, "Techniques for the Study of Speech Pathology," at the ASHA convention in Chicago. Two awards were given, the second to two audiologists and an otologist from Houston for their exhibit showing the otological-audiological team approach to diagnosis and evaluation in restorative hearing surgery. Awards were judged, according to the report in *Asha* (March, 1962, 86-7), "on the basis of excellence of presentation, originality of work, teaching value and whether or not competent, well-informed demonstrators were present the major portion of the time."

The *Asha* description of the Iowa exhibit follows, concluding with this paragraph: "The techniques displayed are being utilized in speech research programs at the University of Iowa and were developed through PHS research grants B-2662 (National Institute of Neurological Diseases and Blindness), D-853 (National Institute of Dental Research), and M-1158 (National Institute of Mental Health), Public Health Service."

At the time the exhibit was prepared and shown, Hardy was supervisor of speech and hearing services at the Hospital School and was an assistant professor in the Department of Speech Pathology and Audiology. Spriestersbach was professor of speech pathology with a joint appointment in the Departments of Speech Pathology and Audiology and Otolaryngology and Maxillofacial Surgery. Moll and Morris were research assistant professors in those two Departments.

THE LANGUAGE OF RESPONSIBILITY

That same year, that is, for the University's 1961 summer session, Johnson was chosen to give the commencement address. He chose to speak on "The Language of Responsibility." The text of his speech was printed in both the August 1961 *Iowa Alumni Review* and the May 1962 *ETC.*

The combination of his humanitarian interest in people with problems, his professional training in speech pathology, and his orientation to general semantics prompted him to include these comments:

As people become more mature they use language more and more responsibly to report accurately what they learn when they listen well and in all other ways observe carefully the facts that are of interest and concern to them. They demonstrate the language of responsibility in describing clearly and in detail what they themselves do that needs to be understood. They speak the language of who, when, where, what and then what, and of the various possible whys, the language of honest and full report and of disciplined explanation—of thoughtful understanding.

Johnson was increasingly in demand as a lecturer in these years, was writing prolifically, and was serving on special committees or as consultant to a variety of professional and governmental agencies. He was, for example, consultant in speech pathology, Walter Reed Army Medical Center, 1954-1961; Central Office consultant in speech pathology, United States Veterans Administration, 1959-1965; consultant to the National Institute of Neurological Diseases and Blindness, 1957; and consultant to the United States Office of Education, 1957-1958; he was on the national advisory council of the Vocational Rehabilitation Administration, 1957-1961; chairman of the section on Vocational Rehabilitation for Handicapped Youth at the White House Conference on Children and Youth, 1960; and a member of the evaluation committee of a special education and rehabilitation study by the Committee on Education and Labor, United States House of Representatives, 1960.

PRESIDENTS CURTIS AND SPRIESTERSBACH

For some months in 1962 the Department included the presidents of two national organizations, Curtis as 1962 president of the American Speech and Hearing Association, Spriestersbach as 1961-1962 president of the American Cleft Palate Assocation.

Curtis, in the three-year period before, during, and immediately following his term of office, was considerably involved in plans for housing the national office. He helped in the investigation of alternatives to the rented space, now outgrown, in downtown Washington, and in his presidential year saw the purchase of the property on which the office was later built. He also worked on the financial plan for funding the construction; it was during his year that the substantial raise in dues, necessary to that plan, was vigorously debated, the debate leading to favorable action the following year.

A major effort in his presidential term brought together the Association and the organization then known as the American Hearing Society, a voluntary agency that supports service programs. Through this effort, the function and purpose of each organization were defined and the appropriate roles of both were clarified to avoid duplication and even conflict of activities.

It was during this time too that Curtis and Raymond Carhart of Northwestern represented the Association and its Education and Training Board through the conferences and discussions with the National Commission on Accrediting, which led to the designation of ASHA in 1962 as the accrediting agency for master's level programs in speech pathology and audiology. That action was by no means a foregone conclusion since, in fact, the NCA had been set up to limit the proliferation of accrediting agencies, not to recognize new ones. In addition, the National Council for Accreditation of Teacher Education as well as the Council for Medical Education and Hospitals was seeking to be named the accrediting agency for this field. And so, Curtis explains, "we had to present a case sufficiently strong that we would not be taken over, so to speak, by one or the other of these groups."

Congress assigned to the Office of Education the legal responsibility for maintaining a list of nationally recognized accrediting agencies, and in 1967 ASHA made the required application to be included on this list. The application was approved August 24 of that year.

Spriestersbach, who had become interested in the American Cleft Palate Association when he first began to teach in the area of organic speech disorders, had served as the ACPA secretary and treasurer from 1957 to 1960. Then, and in his presidential year, just as in his "chief-of-staff service" with Johnson on the Iowa Council, he became known for his ability in organizing, his contributions were to the efficiency as well as the scope of the Association program. (Although the honor came to him a year after the closing date of this Department history, mention may be made here of the fact that he served as Secretary-General of the International Congress on Cleft Palate in Houston, Texas, in 1969.)

CHANGING PATTERNS

In a 1962 Department Report, Curtis writes of the effect of growth on the demand for qualified faculty to staff the developing new programs. "An additional result has been," the Report continues,

> that students seeking careers in this field are now much more widely distributed among the larger number of graduate institutions in which instruction is offered. The fact that the University of Iowa has, nevertheless, continued to attract substantial numbers of qualified graduate students in the field would appear to indicate that it continues to enjoy an excellent reputation and standing.
>
> Another development of recent years concerns the changing patterns of professional service programs in which graduates find

employment. Prior to World War II almost the only clinical services available to persons with language, speech, and hearing handicaps were provided by clinics in universities or clinical programs for school children in a few metropolitan school systems. The public school programs have now spread so that almost any school, except in the more rural areas, offers some services for children with speech and hearing deficiencies. And in recent years there has also been a rapid development of clinical services in speech pathology and audiology in hospitals, community clinics, special treatment centers, and rehabilitation centers. There has thus been both a continuously increasing demand for graduates in the field and a rapid increase in new employment opportunities in hospitals and other special treatment centers. Another increasingly important area of employment for persons with specialized training in speech pathology and audiology, or in speech and hearing science, is as full-time researchers in government research programs, such as that of the National Institute of Dental Research, etc., and in government-supported research programs located in universities.

A few years ago the Ph.D. program in speech pathology and audiology was preparing students for one principal type of position, namely, a college or university post in which the major duties and responsibilities were those of teaching combined with some research and, probably, some clinical duties in a college or university speech and hearing clinic. Now substantial numbers of persons holding Ph.D. degrees are employed as full-time clinicians, or as full-time researchers, possibly also with administrative duties in such programs.

One further trend which should be noted is concerned with the level of education and training required for positions in this field. It is not new, of course, for positions in colleges and universities to require substantial amounts of graduate education. However, until recently many of the clinical services positions in this field have been open to persons with little or no graduate education. In part this resulted from the fact that the field was new and knowledge in the field had not accumulated or been organized; in part, it was a result of the very large demand, in relation to supply, for persons with almost any level of education and training in this special area, so that employers were willing to appoint persons with relatively low levels of training since better trained people were very scarce; and, in part, it resulted from the fact that standards for clinical competence were not well developed. Recently, however, there has been a concerted effort, led by the American Speech and Hearing Association, to raise standards for clinical service in the field and standards of education and training for those who are judged competent to provide such service. Recent changes in the by-laws of the American Speech and Hearing Association provide that, beginning in 1965 a specialized program of graduate study leading to the master's degree, or its equivalent, will be required for either clinical certification by the Assocation or for membership in the Association.

These trends point to greater emphasis on graduate education in the field, greater emphasis on training clinicians even at the Ph.D. level, and greater attention within the clinical services program to the kinds of training that will help prepare students to work in close professional relationships with allied professions such as medicine, dentistry, and clinical psychology.

The courses and degree programs of the Department are planned to meet the needs of students seeking to prepare themselves for a wide variety of career opportunities, including careers as college and university teachers and researchers in speech and hearing disorders and the scientific study of speech and hearing processes and as clinicians in the several clinical settings mentioned above, career objectives that are not mutually exclusive. The offerings also include courses which meet the needs of students with vocational and professional goals in other fields such as psychology, education, speech and dramatic art, dentistry, medicine, etc., whose preparation may be enriched by the study of speech and hearing processes and their disorders.

GRANT SUPPORT

Increase in federal and foundation grant support for both training and teaching was an item of importance throughout the period. The Department could note in the 1962 news release cited above, for example, that

in the past 10 years private foundations and U.S. governmental agencies have granted over one million dollars to SUI for support of research in Speech Pathology and Audiology. In addition, U.S. governmental agencies have been sufficiently impressed with the training program in Speech Pathology and Audiology at SUI that they have granted approximately $580,000 to SUI over a 10-year period in the form of fellowships, traineeships, and related costs of instruction so that more students can receive graduate training in Speech Pathology and Audiology at the University of Iowa.

The Hill Family Foundation, which had supported Johnson's research in stuttering since 1951, continued and increased its support during this period. In 1963 it underwrote his entire salary, and from that time on he carried the title of Louis W. Hill Research Professor.

CHANGES BY 1962

When Curtis wrote the 1962 Department Report, he cited the growing need for reorganization of clinical services, reported a major revision of the curriculum, listed problems related to the Department's inadequate housing, and outlined the strong research program which the faculty had developed by that time.

Service Activities. "The most significant service activities of this Department," he wrote,

> are those which are an integral part of the Department's teaching and research programs, namely, the services rendered through the University Speech Clinic and the other speech pathology and audiology services provided through various University Hospitals departments and related facilities such as the University Hospital School. Only a portion of these is directly supported by the budget of this Department, but all provide service to the State of Iowa and are of vital importance to the teaching and research activities of the Department. Moreover, all are importantly related to the Department's program in that, irrespective of the source of budget support, the professional home base of the persons employed to provide the service is the Department of Speech Pathology and Audiology. This Department has an obligation to coordinate these services, to see that they meet the best possible professional standards, and to provide professional supervision and consultation as needed.
>
> The clinical service activities which are directly supported by the departmental budget include: diagnostic and remedial services in the University Speech Clinic to University students with speech and/or hearing problems; remedial services provided to a limited number of children and adults, not students, who reside in or near Iowa City or who come to Iowa City for the length of time during which service is rendered; diagnostic and counseling services through the Outpatient Speech Clinic; remedial services for selected children of school age by the six-week Summer Speech Clinic Residential Program; diagnostic and remedial services to the public and parochial schools of Iowa City and Coralville, and to the Johnson County special education program.
>
> In addition, programs of speech pathology and audiology services include the following:
>
> (a) Diagnostic and counseling services as needed to all patients seen in the Department of Otolaryngology and Maxillofacial Surgery. These services are provided by a staff paid largely from the funds of that department and supervised by Spriestersbach and Prather whose salaries are shared by that Department and the Department of Speech Pathology and Audiology.
>
> (b) Diagnostic and consultative services as needed for patients seen in the Department of Pediatrics and the Child Development Clinic. The personnel providing these services are paid from funds from the United States Bureau made available through the State Services for Crippled Children.
>
> (c) Diagnostic, consultative, and limited remedial services to

patients seen in the Department of Neurology and the Division of Neurosurgery and in the Hospital School Rehabilitation Unit. This service program has been developed in recent years. It provides mainly for patients with aphasic and dysarthric symptoms due to neurological damage. The staff to provide these services is furnished by the Department of Speech Pathology and Audiology.

(d) Speech and hearing services in the University Hospital School. The school employs a staff for this service consisting of six full-time and one half-time professional people and a full-time secretary. The supervisor of this service is Hardy who also teaches courses in the Department and a portion of whose salary is paid by this Department.

(e) Diagnostic services provided through the Mobile Clinics of the State Services for Crippled Children. Staff for this service is provided from U.S. Children's Bureau funds made available through State Services for Crippled Children.

(f) Speech pathology and audiology services in the Iowa City Veterans Administration Hospital. Currently the Hospital pays the salary of a half-time audiologist. Speech pathology services are provided through a cooperative arrangement with the Department. The staff member primarily responsible for these services is Luther F. Sies who works directly with patients and also supervises the clinic work of students enrolled in practicum courses.

In addition, individual staff members provide other services to the state: Curtis, Hast, Prather, and Smith serve as members of the Iowa Committee for the Conservation of Hearing, a committee of the state Department of Health which meets regularly three or four times each year; Sherman and Jordan are on the advisory committee on speech correction services of the Division of Special Education of the State Department of Public Instruction. Hardy serves as a consultant to the Cedar Rapids Cerebral Palsy Center.

Interdepartmental and intercollege relationships are deeply involved in both the research and clinical services programs. They have evolved because of mutual interests and needs but they have become extremely complex and, in a very real sense, unwieldy. With respect to the clinical services program especially the relations are most complicated. Williams has the title of Director of the University Speech Clinic. However, if he confined the scope of his activities to those services which are provided by the University Speech Clinic, per se, he would have little or nothing to do with a large part of the speech and hearing services provided through the various programs described in the previous section. It seems apparent that an administrative reorganization of the clinical services program is overdue. This is needed not only to provide a more unified and coordinated structure but, even more importantly, to provide students with improved and more comprehensive clinical training experiences and to better serve the research program. . . .

It is recommended that a staff of persons with full-time clinical responsibilities be employed on a 12-month basis in sufficient number to provide these [clinical] services [including eventually, it is hoped, a residential clinic], to have primary responsibility for the welfare of the client but also to cooperate in the professional training of students in such ways as supervising students enrolled for practicums and lecturing to students and medical residents. They will also be expected to participate in research projects as well as in workshops for parents and consultations with speech and hearing clinicians throughout the state. It is recommended that a position entitled Director of Clinical Services in Speech Pathology and Audiology be created to supersede the present position of Director of the University Speech Clinic.

Curriculum Revision. The program for undergraduate majors, Curtis pointed out,

has been undergoing revision and is currently in a transitional stage. Formerly the majority of undergraduate students in the department were enrolled in the program terminating in the B.A. and designed to qualify them for positions as speech correctionists or speech and hearing specialists in public school programs. This curriculum also met the academic requirements of the Basic Clinical Certificate of the American Speech and Hearing Association. This was necessarily a rather rigidly prescribed program in order to provide the necessary professional courses in speech pathology as well as the courses in educational psychology, educational philosophy, and methods required by the state educational certifying agencies. A smaller number of students, who planned to continue their professional education through one or more years of graduate study before seeking jobs followed a more flexible and less completely prescribed curriculum.

In part, because of trends and developments described above but also because the faculty of this Department has for a number of years believed that adequate preparation of a specialist in this field requires a substantial amount of graduate level study, *the Department has recently reorganized its curricula to provide for an integrated program of undergraduate and graduate study in which the lowest terminal degree for persons seeking employment as clinical specialists in this field will be the M.A. degree.* [Italics ours.] During an interim period, students who will complete their undergraduate program prior to June 1965 will be permitted to elect the old four-year degree program leading to a bachelor's degree and certification as public school speech correctionists.

The curriculum leading to the bachelor of science degree in speech pathology and audiology is described in the 1962 University catalogue as "the undergraduate portion of an integrated curriculum leading to a terminal M.A. degree with clinical emphasis." The curriculum leading to the bachelor of arts degree in speech pathology and audiology "provides a major for students wishing to concentrate on studies of language, speech, and hearing problems as part of a four-year liberal arts program; it also provides preparation for students planning graduate study leading to the Ph.D. degree in speech and hearing science, or in speech pathology and audiology. This curriculum provides considerably greater flexibility in planning a program of studies than does that that leads to the B.S. degree."

Curtis, some six years later, commented on the thinking that had gone into this new terminal M.A. program which was in effect at Iowa a year before ASHA moved in the same direction, that is, to require the M.A. for membership and certification after 1965. "We had felt the need for this kind of a change much before the national Association took action," Curtis explains.

> We felt we could not really, with a four-year degree, provide anything like an adequate professional education without so sacrificing the basic liberal education of the student that we were unjustified in the four-year pattern. We had serious discussions. We asked ourselves whether we, as one university, could act in isolation to change this, could strike out on our own and do this kind of thing when everybody else was doing something different. Philosophically our belief was that this was a direction in which we had to go, in which everybody had to go. And we wanted to move as rapidly as we could. But there were practical considerations too. This was a pragmatic matter. And so we did not move as rapidly as our beliefs and convictions would have taken us. But long before the time we felt we could make a formal announcement we were advising students, unless there were compelling reasons that prevented their doing this, to think immediately about going on for not less than a master's degree.

Space Problems. Instructional rooms, Curtis pointed out in his 1962 Report,

> are primarily located in East Hall and are shared with other departments and teaching programs; occasionally large lecture courses are taught elsewhere. Room C314, the only room used for class meetings that is not assigned through the Registrar's Office, serves as a small classroom; seminar room; demonstration room for lab sections in voice and phonetics, fundamentals of hearing, and psychoacoustics; laboratory for the course in laboratory instrumentation; teaching and laboratory room for classes in speech reading; and for group clinical work in speech reading. It has been especially equipped for certain of these uses.
> Office space is at a premium with a number of staff members sharing offices. Offices are scattered: in East Hall, the University Hospitals, and the Hospital School.
> The laboratory in E-11 East Hall was constructed in 1950 and was

adequate at the time but now, with expansion of both the research program and the teaching program using this space, there are serious scheduling problems and frequent conflicts between the programs.

By the use of prefabricated soundproof booths, laboratory spaces have been provided in two small rooms in C312, East Hall. With the space used for laboratories, it is not available for clinical services and so the already crowded clinic room situation becomes more critical.

Laboratory spaces outside of East Hall include the cineradiographic laboratory in the research wing of University Hospitals and the Speech Respiration Laboratory in the Hospital School, already mentioned. They are well equipped but their location makes it difficult to use them fully in teaching, for demonstrations, etc.

The most significant statement that can be made concerning our present facilities is that they are inadequate, from the point of square-footage available, for all uses: office, laboratory, clinic, storage. They are also scattered and extremely inefficient from the standpoint of location. This situation will become worse when the Gables [a former residence, on Dubuque Street] is razed to make room for the Zoology Building addition. [The Gables was razed later that year and the Clinic moved to two University-owned houses on Melrose Avenue.]

It is recommended that a Speech and Hearing Services Center be established in close proximity to University Hospitals and that the Center shall be housed in a new speech pathology and audiology building to be constructed at the earliest feasible date. The Center shall provide a year-round program of speech pathology and audiology services to maintain a coordinated service and referral program for University Hospitals patients who are in need of such services. Existing services already established within the hospital departments shall continue to be carried on in those departments under the direction of the appropriate department head or other officer to the extent that such operation will contribute to the overall efficiency of service to the patient. Longer-term remedial services of a nonmedical nature will be provided in the Center under policies to be established. The Center will also provide other diagnostic and remedial services currently provided by the University Speech Clinic, the Outpatient Speech Clinic, and the Summer Speech Clinic Residential Program. It will also provide the services required by a residential program for children if and when establishment of such a residential program becomes possible.

More immediate than space needs in a new building is our need for space until such a building can become a reality. We are in desperate need for office space, clinic space, and laboratory space. An interim provision must be made.

Research. Progress is reported in the research programs of Johnson and Williams, Sherman, Small, and Spriestersbach, described in the 1960 Report. These three items are among others included in the 1962 Report:

Grants from the National Institute of Dental Research have provided the equipment for a cineradiographic laboratory located in the research wing of University Hospitals. This equipment is being utilized for fundamental studies of physiology of speech articulation, for the research program on cleft palate, and for research in music, as well as for diagnostic examinations.

Most recently a significant research program concerned with respiratory physiology in relation to speech has been developed in cooperation between the Department and the University Hospital School. This is supported by a grant to the School from the National Institute for Neurological Diseases and Blindness. The program is broad in concept and is engaged in investigating respiratory function in normal speech as well as in the speech of individuals with neuromuscular disorders. Work in the area had begun before the grant period with two Ph.D. dissertations completed under the direction of Curtis. The grant supports personnel but also provides for a major share of equipment for a well-equipped laboratory located in the School which will make possible full utilization of electromyographic, spirometric, and other observational techniques in the study of respiratory function in speech. This program and the program of research utilizing the cineradiographic techniques complement each other in a particularly significant way.

Prior to his resignation Darley had developed a significant research program concerned with language development in children and disturbances of language functions, such as aphasia. This program of research is being continued, with at least three Ph.D. studies in progress. The helpful cooperation of staff members from the Psychology Department should be acknowledged in relation to these studies as well as in other phases of the research program.

Then Curtis adds at the end of this section:

Of particular note in relation to research and creative activity is the outstanding work that Sherman has been doing as Editor of the *Journal of Speech and Hearing Research* since 1959. As the *first editor* of this new publication of the American Speech and Hearing Association she deserves major credit for the fact that from the beginning it has been a journal of high quality and in three years has achieved widespread recognition as a major research journal in the field of speech and hearing science.

STATE FUNDS FOR BUILDING

In 1963 Iowa's Sixtieth General Assembly appropriated $750,000 in state funds for the construction of the Department's new building on a site at the west edge of the University's medical center. Plans for the building had been received from the architects more than a year earlier and were now being discussed by the faculty with representatives of government agencies with a view to obtaining matching federal funds. Later an additional $340,000 was voted by the state for equipment for the building, and it was hoped that this too would be augmented by federal grants.

1963 CONFERENCES

Participation in conferences, on the campus and away, was a continuing activity for faculty members during this period, as it had been in preceding periods. In 1963, for example, Spriestersbach was Conference Committee chairman for the ASHA Conference on Graduate Education in Speech Pathology at Highland Park, April 29-May 3, and was principal investigator for the conference on Cleft Lip and Palate, Criteria for Physical Management, on the Iowa campus October 28-30. The former meeting was supported by a grant from the National Institute of Neurological Diseases and Blindness, and the latter by the National Institute of Dental Research. Johnson was a member of the ASHA Research Committee which planned the Highland Park Conference, Darley was editor of the conference, Curtis and Williams were participants, as were Strother, Schubert, Parker, and Fairbanks, formerly of the Iowa faculty. Of the 106 attending, 33 had their highest degrees from Iowa.

Morris was editor of the Cleft Palate Conference and Moll did one of the three orientation papers. Darley and Melrose were participants, and Moll and Jeanne K. Smith were recorders.

1964

Curtis notes in the 1964 Department Report that with the substantial increase in emphasis on graduate education, "practically all students seeking careers in the field have the master's degree as the minimum goal. There is an increased emphasis on professional clinical training, even at the Ph.D. level, since the trends in the demand for professional services require this level of graduate education for many clinical positions."

He notes two "developments of significance" since the 1962 report:

(a) The Department was awarded a Training Grant from the National Institute of Neurological Diseases and Blindness effective September 1963, to support a number of predoctoral and postdoctoral traineeships, as well as certain parts of the teaching program.

(b) A Speech Pathology and Audiology Clinic has been established in the Iowa City Veterans Administration Hospital with a current staff of two full-time Ph.D.-level people. This program provides traineeships for graduate students, usually doctoral candidates. New quarters are to be provided and an expanded program is indicated by the VA Central Office. This program provides additional support for doctoral candidates preparing for professional clinical careers and also an additional service facility through which the practicum experiences of students in the Department may be broadened.

Clinic Needs. "The need continues," he emphasizes,

for a full-time clinical staff to strengthen teaching in practicum courses and to carry part of the clinical service load, as stressed in previous reports.

Over the years, as the teaching program in speech and hearing disorders has developed, the pattern of organization of responsibilities which has developed is as follows: Each of the several full-time faculty responsible for teaching the clinical courses has developed a special area of interest and in that area is responsible for teaching substantive courses and seminars, for carrying on research and directing graduate programs, for teaching practicum courses, and for clinical work with patients whose problems lie in that area. Graduate assistants have been assigned to help them. As the programs have increased, these assistants have become more and more involved in ways that are not appropriate to their levels of training and experience. The obvious solution would appear to be additions of full-time staff to handle many of the clinical duties. We are asking for a beginning to made during the next biennium by the addition of one such person.

New Building. Applications have been made, Curtis reports, for "federal construction grants for the new building but so far no action has been taken."

Meanwhile the quarters in East Hall were becoming even more of a problem than they had been before. An addition for Psychology laboratories was being constructed inside the "U" and across the front of the building, which meant that building activity and piles of building materials literally surrounded the offices and laboratories in the ground floor east wing. Curtis asked the administration for air conditioners because "it would be impossible to have windows open during the phases of construction that create dust and dirt and equally impossible to work during warm weather with the windows closed." Air conditioners were forthcoming for most of the rooms affected.

A MEMORABLE 1965

The year 1965 was eventful in several ways. That year Wendell Johnson died. That same year the construction contract was let for the speech and hearing center he and many others had worked for so hard and so long. That year, the Department restructured its clinical services program and sent recommendations to Dean Stuit for a new undergraduate major in speech science. And that year Spriestersbach was president of ASHA and was appointed Dean of the Iowa Graduate College.

Interestingly enough, Spriestersbach's accension to the deanship completed—within the Curtis period—an unusually inclusive change of administrative personnel in those areas most closely associated with the Program's interdisciplinary activities. Since the personnel changes are part of the background for the year, they will be considered first here.

PERSONNEL CHANGES BY 1965

Changes in administrative personnel in associated areas began the first year of the Department, that is, in 1956. Clay Harshbarger that year became head of the Department of Speech and Dramatic Arts, following the death of E. C. Mabie. The same year, Dr. Paul Huston was named director of the Psychopathic Hospital and head of the Department of Psychiatry to succeed Dr. Wilbur Miller, who had succeeded Dr. Andrew Woods, who had succeeded Dr. Thomas Brennan, who had succeeded Dr. Samuel Orton of the Travis period.

In 1960 Boyd McCandless resigned and was succeeded by Charles Spiker as director of the Child Welfare Research Station, which in 1963 became the Institute of Child Behavior and Development. In 1960 Dean Walter F. Loehwing of the Graduate College died and was succeeded by Ralph Shriner, acting dean for several weeks, Stow Persons, acting dean 1960-1961, John Weaver, dean 1961-1964, and Orville Hitchcock, acting dean, 1964-1965.

In 1962 Mark Hale was succeeded by Frank Glick as director of the School of Social Work, and E. T. Peterson was succeeded by Howard Jones as Dean of the College of Education.

In 1963, Dr. Dean Lierle, head of the Department of Otolaryngology and Maxillofacial Surgery retired and was succeeded by Dr. Brian McCabe. Dr. Lierle had worked closely with the Program for more than thirty-five years, almost as long as Mabie had, coming into it actively when he was named head of his Department in 1928, and continuing so since then. He had given his own time and effort, and had also made the time and effort of Scott Reger available to the Program.

In 1964 University President Virgil M. Hancher retired and was succeeded by Howard R. Bowen who, like Hancher, had had special contact with the Iowa Program. President Hancher had served through a quarter century of its development, in the Strother and Johnson as well as the Curtis periods. President Bowen had been aware of the Program both as a student and as a faculty member in earlier years at Iowa, then had further contact with the new discipline through Iowa's Grant Fairbanks, whom he came to know well when he and Fairbanks were colleagues on the University of Illinois faculty.

Also in 1964, Kenneth Spence resigned as chairman of the Psychology Department, and a year later was succeeded by Judson Brown. Leonard Eron was acting chairman in the interim.

ASHA PRESIDENT, 1965

When Spriestersbach became ASHA president in 1965, his administration had the responsibility of working with the architects in planning the design of the national headquarters office in Washington. The project had been developed with the approval of the ASHA membership. "The design we finally chose was something Kenneth Johnson, our executive secretary, pushed for and I supported him very strongly," Spriestersbach explains. "I think we have a very useful building. At the same time it is a beautiful building and one with which I think we can identify with pride."

During his year as president, Spriestersbach made an effort to improve communication within the membership as a whole, one such effort being his monthly "As I See It" column in *Asha*. He felt he had "an amazing amount of feedback" from this.

Characteristically, he made contributions to the ordering of things during his term in office. Among these was the initiation of a practice, that has continued since, of including a "whereas" statement as part of all motions of the Council, so that when Council proceedings are published the reader can have some notion of the context in which action was being taken. This was obviously another effort to improve communication.

DEAN SPRIESTERSBACH, 1965

Spriestersbach retained his appointment in the Department when he became Dean of the Graduate College. He continued to do a limited amount of teaching there although his main base from then on was in the University administration as Dean and, from 1966, also as Vice-President for Research.

In his accession to the deanship lies a curious turn of history. Through his appointment the Program once again had an unusually close tie with the Graduate College, a tie that dates back to the days when Seashore, Dean of that College and head of the Psychology Department first used his creative genius to initiate the graduate-training regimen out of which the Iowa Program and the Department of Speech Pathology and Audiology eventually grew. Seashore was Dean from 1908 to 1936. After him came George Stoddard, another great friend of the Program, who was Dean from 1936 to 1942, and who was followed by Seashore, who came out of retirement to serve for four war years.

Thus, beginning the year of Travis' Ph.D. and continuing through to the end of the Curtis period, the Deanship has been held twenty-five of the forty-four years by a man with a significant professional interest in the Program. A less conservative figure would be twenty-nine years out of forty-eight, if C. C. Bunch's Ph.D. in 1920 were considered the beginning, or even thirty-five years out of fifty-three, going back to 1915, when Seashore is said to have conceived the general notion from which the Iowa Program emerged.

REORGANIZATION, 1965

The reorganization of clinical services provided the long-sought revision of administrative structure in the clinic area and the addition of full-time professional clinical personnel there, as Curtis had recommended year after year in his Department Reports.

With the reorganization, the chief administrative officer in the clinic area became the Director of Clinical Services, this title superseding that of Director of the Speech Clinic. (So there was no longer the title of Director of the Speech Clinic. Travis was the first to hold it, in 1927; then it passed in turn to Strother, Johnson, Darley, and, most recently, to Williams. Its use within the Iowa Program had spanned thirty-eight years, and its use by Seashore in Psychology had preceded that.)

The reorganization plan *(7)* designated the Director's assistant as the Clinic Coordinator, a position already in existence, and his full-time staff as Clinical Supervisors. Their positions were newly defined. In brief, duties were as follows: the *Director of Clinical Services* is responsible for carrying out policies set by the Department, attends to top-level administrative work of the Clinic, monitors ongoing clinical activities, and keeps the total Department faculty informed of these. The *Clinic Coordinator* takes care of clinical services records and scheduling, and files of the Department and between the Department and other Departments and agencies; checks with the Director on the agenda for meetings; makes sure that "everything gets done that has to be done." All clients of the Clinic are assigned to a *Clinical Supervisor* who is then responsible for that client, and who directly supervises any student's work with the client. The *Clinical Supervisor* must have an advanced degree in the field, must hold an ASHA certificate of clinical competence, and must have had clinical experience. He or she has full faculty status, and promotions are in the regular academic line.

By adding Clinical Superivisors so qualified, the Department was filling the long-felt need for strengthening the clinical training program in that direction. Beyond that, however—and some have suggested that this was as important—by adding Clinical Supervisors as members of the faculty, the Department was for the first time giving official recognition to the teaching role of such personnel. The formalizing of this recognition within the University structure followed discussions that Curtis had in 1965, first with Dean Stuit, then with Dean Stuit and Dean Willard L. Boyd, Vice-President for Academic Affairs and Dean of Faculties, who succeeded Howard Bowen as President of the University in 1968. In these discussions, Curtis simply pointed out that these Supervisors were indeed teaching, that "a program of clinical training must have a laboratory in which people learn to work with people, with their problems, and they must be supervised adequately. And this is a very, very important teaching function in this kind of program. So these people are just as much a part of the teaching faculty as anyone else and they ought to have open to them the same opportunities for promotion and recognition as anyone else." Neither Dean Stuit nor Dean Boyd seriously disagreed with this point of view, as Curtis recalls, but the discussions were a necessary step in the process of clarifying the relation of clinical work to other work in the Department following the reorganization.

The Clinic's adjunct faculty continued to be composed of those members of the faculty whose principal work was in teaching and/or research, but who spent a considerable amount of time supervising the clinical work of students. (At the end of the Curtis period this adjunct faculty included Fisher, Hardy, Melrose, Sherman, and Williams, in the Department; Anderson, Morris, and Duane Van Demark, jointly in the Department and in Otolaryngology; Ann Van Demark, jointly in the Department and the Veterans Administration; and Herbert Jordan with the Veterans Administration.)

Melrose was named the first Director of Clinical Services, and served in that capacity from 1965 through the remainder of the Curtis period; Bette Spriestersbach had been serving as Clinic Coordinator since 1963, continued in that position through the period, and then was succeeded by Jan Whitebook; Elaine Dripps, Marie Emge, Aaron Favors, Linda Smith Jordan, and Judith Milisen Knabe became Clinical Supervisors.

In the reorganization plan, the Clinic gained a social work division as part of the Clinic structure. This division was directed by a professional supervisor of social work (the position during the Curtis period was held by Barbara Moeller), who had as her staff graduate students of the School of Social Work who were getting field training in social work during their service on her staff.

A related matter, and one which in 1968 was still under study as it had been for most of the period, was the possibility of the establishment of a year-round residential speech and hearing clinic. This, it was felt, would round out the Department's total facilities for clinical practicum work by providing students with an opportunity to work with clients through longer term rehabilitative procedures than are feasible without a residential facility.

REORGANIZATION: THE SUMMER CLINIC

Until the reorganization of the administrative structure of clinical services in 1965 the Summer Clinic had been an adjunct of the regular program, with its own special staff and director. Thus while Williams was Director of the Clinic from the beginning of the period until 1965, Darley was Director of the Summer Clinic until 1962, and Evan Jordan for the summers of 1963 and 1964. Delta Falvey, who as a social worker had been supervisor of the social service unit of the foster care agency serving all of the University clinics, became the social worker for the summer residential program in 1955. She continued in that position until 1965.

With the 1965 reorganization, by becoming Director of Clinical Services, Melrose was not only Director of the Clinic but also Director of the Summer Clinic, and his newly organized staff served with him. This plan was made to provide a more coherent continuing program than was possible before.

Summer activities moved with the Clinic itself in 1962 from East Hall and the Gables to a University-owned house on Melrose Avenue. In 1967 they were moved to the new Speech and Hearing Center. As had been the case for some years, children at the Summer Clinic lived in a fraternity house and came to the Clinic for therapy, usually two or three or four hours a day.

By 1968 the Summer Clinic program involved from eight to ten resident counselors who were graduate students or seniors. They lived with the fifty children for the six-week period and contributed to the recreation program scheduled at the end of each day. There was also a supporting household staff to take care of the details of day-to-day living. Counselors were given a week's orientation before the clinic opened.

The Director of Clinical Services, the Clinic Coordinator, and the Clinical Supervisors function as the professional staff. Each takes his assigned share of the responsibility for the administration, the coordination, the direct clinical work with the children who come, and the orientation of counselors.

CONTRACT LETTING, 1965

Contracts for the construction of the new Speech and Hearing Center were let by the Board of Regents in August 1965. The totals for construction and equipment were just in excess of two million dollars. The total for construction was $1,521,000, of which $750,000 was from state funds and $771,000 was in grants from government agencies. The total for equipment was $492,000, of which $340,000 was from state funds and $152,000 in grants from government agencies. Construction began that fall.

Wendell Johnson, 1906-1965

Wendell Johnson, who in these years had been amazingly active in spite of his illness of 1954-55, was once again slowed by his heart problem in March 1963, but even so managed to teach a few classes, to counsel, to lecture, and to write. Characteristically, he was writing longhand on his clipboard (a contribution on "speech disorders" for the *Encyclopaedia Britannica*) when he died on August 29, 1965.

His death was noted, and his work chronicled widely, in the metropolitan press and national news magazines, as well as in many scholarly journals. The tribute in *Asha* was written by his colleagues on the Iowa faculty. Memorial numbers were issued by *ETC.* (September 1968) and the *General Semantics Bulletin* (No. 32 and 33, 1965/1966).

Many of his friends cherished especially the tribute written by his long-time colleague and former student, Dean Spriestersbach, a part of which appeared in the August 31, 1965, *Iowa City Press Citizen:*

> It is difficult for me to comment on the life of Wendell Johnson because he was my teacher, mentor, and great, good friend. And while I was privileged to know him and to work with him for more than 25 years, my feelings are not unique. For he was teacher, mentor, and great, good friend of literally hundreds of other persons throughout the world.
>
> The results of his life's work are a matter of record. It is one of prolific writing, lecturing, consulting, advising. It is a record which reveals a man with imagination, idealism, and optimism; a man with a contempt for complacency, cynicism, and lethargy. It is a record to which many men aspire but few achieve.
>
> Wendell Johnson was one of the truly great professors that a university is privileged to have. He argued consistently for the philosophy that knowledge could not be packaged and claimed by departments and colleges. In fact, he startled many college and university administrators by questioning the validity of what, to him, were arbitrary academic units which tended to inhibit the solution of problems because they fostered a kind of academic provincialism.
>
> But, in my view, his greatness is to be found in the impact he had on people. He inspired and stimulated them. He caused them, sometimes almost in spite of themselves, to become something more than they could have without his influence. He gave smiles and pats-on-the-back freely and sincerely. . . . Wendell Johnson will be missed but he has left a heritage which will never be forgotten.

O. R. Bontrager, Johnson's fellow student at Iowa forty years before, and later a university professor, included these words in his tribute in the memorial issue of the *General Semantics Bulletin:*

To those who knew him, these words must appear as an anti-climax. To those who did not, no words could possibly portray him. He would have laughed at the thought that anyone should ever call him "great."

His genuine human warmth came through no matter what words he spoke. He was utterly devoid of pomposity. . . . Never did he reveal a trace of arrogance. A man of great integrity, he could be counted on. He lived what he advocated. His relationships with others were never weakened by delusions of his own omnipotence and grandeur.

Students came to hear him from all over the world. Hundreds of them will long remember how rare was their good fortune to have known him. My own debt to him is very great. . . . [His] life will always stand out as a model of the humanity we must eventually achieve if we are to measure up to the test of continued existence.

CURRICULUM REVISION, 1965

In his 1966 Department Report, Curtis recounted that in October 1965 the Department had submitted recommendations for its second major revision of curricula and course offerings. "The principal changes in the new curricula are concerned," he pointed out,

with the program of undergraduate studies and with the curricula leading to a professional master's degree in either speech pathology or audiology.

These changes reflect the fact that within recent years there has been a rapid development in certain fields of scientific inquiry related to an understanding of human oral communication processes, *e.g.*, physiological and acoustic phonetics, psychoacoustics, linguistics, and psycholinguistics. It is the belief of this faculty that a person who is preparing himself to understand and cope with disorders of human communication must have a reasonable grasp of information and concepts in these fields as well as an adequate background in certain other related fields, such as psychology, anatomy of the speech and hearing mechanisms, etc. Study in these areas requires, furthermore, a more adequate background in mathematics and in natural science, especially physics and biology, than we have heretofore required of undergraduate students.

To implement this fundamental philosophy concerning what we regard as sound professional education in speech pathology and audiology, *an undergraduate major in speech science has been instituted.* [Italics ours.] It will replace the old undergraduate major in speech pathology and audiology which contained a substantial body of courses dealing with disorders of speech, hearing, and language. In contrast, the curriculum in speech and hearing science provides for a concentration of studies embracing the fields previously mentioned. No courses of a professional nature concerned with disorders of speech, hearing, and language are required for the bachelor's degree, although a few such courses may be elected in the senior year. Consistent with this philosophy, the master's degree curricula in speech pathology and in audiology have been revised to include certain courses of a professional nature formerly taught as part of the undergraduate curriculum.

The advantages of these curricula changes are believed to be the following:

(a) The undergraduate Program in speech and hearing science provides a much improved preparation for graduate study for those interested in the clinical areas of speech, hearing, and language disorders. With this preparation as background the professional courses can be taught much more effectively, with both a scope and depth that is not possible with students whose previous preparation is less adequate.

(b) The undergraduate program in speech and hearing science also provides, and for the first time, an adequate base on which to build a program of graduate studies for the person whose primary interest is in speech and hearing science, per se.

(c) We believe (at least we sincerely hope) that this program will attract a high level of student who may be led into this field because of an intellectual curiosity concerning the fundamental nature of human communication and the disorders thereof.

(d) As previously indicated, we believe this program is consistent with recent developments of knowledge in the areas related to human oral communication and represents a logical sequence of studies that should lead to development of high levels of competence for both professional clinical workers and research scholars.

SHIFTS AFTER CURRICULUM REVISION

With the increased emphasis on graduate work there was not only an increase in the number of graduate degrees granted, but also the expected shrinkage in total number of undergraduate majors after the terminal M.A. program had been introduced in 1962, and again after the M.A. requirement went into effect nationally in 1965.

The Department's enrollment, by degree programs, has been:

Year	B.S., B.A.	M.A.	Ph.D.
1956-57	not available	*	*
1957-58	81	**	**
1958-59	92	21	15
1959-60	106	25	21

Year	B.S., B.A.	M.A.	Ph.D.
1960-61	101	29	18
1961-62	125	40	15
1962-63	134	40	15
1963-64	124	48	20
1964-65	129	43	24
1965-66	107	57	26
1966-67	101	49	28
1967-68	80	53	25

*Total of 39 in graduate work; breakdown not available

**Total of 43 in graduate work; breakdown not available

It is to be understood that because all degrees before 1956 were in "something else," this listing of totals must be regarded as approximate, but on the side of understatement. Totals given here are supported by official records but may be incomplete. If the first degree counted is Travis's M.A. in 1923, then the total number of graduate degrees from that beginning to 1956, the year of the Department, is 256 M.A.s and 134 Ph.D.s; from the beginning to 1962, the year of the curriculum revision, is 364 M.A.s and 158 Ph.D.s; and from the beginning through June 1968 is 485 M.A.s and 194 Ph.D.s.

EDUCATION FOR THE DEAF

The University's training program in education for the deaf was considerably revised about this time (the midsixties) by Clifford E. Howe of the College of Education after conferences with a number of people, including Fisher and Curtis. As of the spring of 1968 the revision had been accomplished, grant support was being sought, and recruitment of a qualified administrator was in progress.

The original program had emerged soon after Curtis became head of the Department. It was the product of his effort and the efforts of Superintendent Lloyd E. Berg and Principal (now Superintendent) C. Joseph Giangreco of the School for the Deaf at Council Bluffs, and James Stroud of the College of Education, now retired. These men had concluded that the program should be in the College of Education, not the

Department, since its purpose was to train classroom teachers to teach subject matter to deaf children, not speech clinicians to be classroom teachers. Howe, who in 1966 became chairman of the recently created division of special education in the College of Education, has retained that central purpose in the revision.

OUT OF EAST HALL

When it came time, in the fall of 1967, to move from East Hall into the handsome new red brick building which was to be known as the Wendell Johnson Speech and Hearing Center, many found that their pleasure in going into the fine new quarters was tempered a bit by the feeling that they were leaving home. They were, of course, in a way. Those East Hall rooms to which the Program had come in its infancy had seen the trials and frustrations and joys of thirty-seven years of growth and change, had seen the Program become a Council and then a Department, had seen Seashore and Travis, Strother and Stoddard, Mabie and Johnson, and so many others come and go. The old building was crowded, certainly, and ill-suited to current needs. But it was graced by memories.

The move, with the inevitable mountains of boxes and the puzzlements of what goes where, was considerably more than a simple building-to-building shift. East Hall was not the only place involved, for during the period the Department had expanded until it was sheltered by several roofs, but East Hall's was the largest. Under that roof there were the third floor center rooms and the rooms on the ground floor of the east wing that had been used since 1930. Then there was a suite of rooms on the third floor of the east wing, in use since 1957, principally as offices of the *Journal of Speech and Hearing Research* when Sherman was editor of that publication. There was also space in the barracks east of East Hall, occupied since the late forties. There were two University houses on Melrose Avenue, in use by the Clinic and people of the Clinic staff since 1962 when they had to vacate the offices in the Gables. And, in addition to all these, there were individual offices scattered throughout the hospital complex.

So the first weeks of the fall of 1967 were times of confusion and mixed emotions. There was a certain amount of merriment too, as Department personnel discovered who else worked there—after all, this was the first time since World War II that everyone had been housed in the same building. Once the newness of the surroundings could be accommodated to, many found that the legacy of the past had not been left behind after all, but had come over from East Hall and was settling in just as they were.

CERTIFICATION AGAIN

It was pleasant for Curtis to recall recently the climate in which the State of Iowa revised its certification requirements for speech clinicians by setting the minimum after July 1, 1968, as the master's degree level of preparation. This of course followed the similar change in the national requirement.

He feels it is worth noting that "by this time we had a great deal of support within the State Department of Public Instruction," a situation differing considerably from the one he faced in 1947, when as the first president of the new Iowa Speech Correction Association, he and his colleagues began their long struggle for a certification program in Iowa. At that time there was only one person in the state with certification, Dorothy Sherman.

In the sixties, however, in contrast,

> the people within the Division of Special Education were highly supportive of us in attempting to get this kind of change brought about. And the change was recommended by an advisory committee that was called by the State Department itself, almost a reversal of the previous situation. So it can be said that this change (in the sixties) was recommended by people in the field, who were most knowledgeable about the field, and not imposed from above. This was really quite a change.

Iowa, he notes, traditionally has had a national leadership role in state public school correction programs. He feels that the Iowa faculty and their students have made a large contribution to this, joining many others in a sustained effort over a long period of time. Much has been done since the Travis era, when there were almost no openings for speech correctionists in Iowa schools. Much was done during the years of the Curtis period. As late as 1956, according to an item in the ISHA *Therapist* for February of that year, there were then no speech clinicians in the schools of forty-three of Iowa's ninety-nine counties. In the remaining fifty-six counties there was a total of sixty-two. As of 1968 there were 235 in Iowa public schools. Every county has "some speech services within its boundaries or is attempting to locate speech clinicians who provide these services," according to the Department of Public Instruction *(13)*.

CLINICAL SERVICES

The scope of clinical services in the Department at the end of the Curtis period is suggested in this summary by Melrose *(7)*, the Director:

> At any given time we have between 100 and 120 clients who are being seen on a regular basis, that is to say, one, two, or three appointments

a week. We also see three or four people a week on outpatient day which at the present time is a Wednesday. At that time we have a complete workup for any client who comes in. This means a speech, hearing, and otolaryngological examination, psychological workup, social work interviews, conferences with other professional people, and conferences with parents, so that decisions can be made as to what the problem is and what can be done about it. This is an ongoing program, operating about 40 weeks out of the year, in which we see three or four people weekly for outpatient evaluation.

We are responsible for speech and hearing screening of the University's freshmen and transfer students. And this amounts to three or four thousand examinations a year. And in the summer clinic we have about 50 children each year.

As a staff and as individuals on the staff, we also are involved in consultation with other agencies who ask for help. We are involved with the Head Start Program, doing the speech and hearing screening and the language testing for 50 children here full-time for the Program. We are involved with such things as the Migrant Workers Program where hearing testing is needed. And we are becoming involved with the Regional Educational Services Administration, a four-county administration for special services in education which fits into Iowa's growing program of intercooperative multicounty units, eventually leading to a 16-area statewide plan for medical services, special services for school children, educational services, and so on.

Students in our Department receive some part of their clinical practicum training in the Speech and Hearing Clinic under the direction of the Clinical Supervisors. They also do some part of their practicum work in the Department of Otolaryngology and Maxillofacial Surgery, the Department of Pediatrics, and the Department of Neurology, in the College of Medicine, at the Veterans Administration facility, in the public and parochial schools of Iowa City and Coralville, in the University Hospital School, the Pine School for retarded children, in the Child Development Clinic, in the Oakdale Rehabilitation Center, and with State Services for Crippled Children and Adults.

Speech and hearing work goes on in each of these agencies. And our students go to these agencies for training either in clinical practicum work or in diagnostic workups of the clients who come to those agencies for diagnosis and/or therapy.

One of the responsibilities of the Director of Clinical Services is to maintain liaison between all these agencies and the Department. Meetings of representatives of the agencies and the Department are held from time to time to discuss problems and projects. The important thing is to maintain a close working relationship between all the people involved.

THE INTERDISCIPLINARY EMPHASIS

In his 1966 Department Report, Curtis had put the work in context with these words:

A major feature of the Department's program which has been stated in previous reports but which cannot be over-emphasized is the interdepartmental and interdisciplinary nature of the Program. Aside from the course preparation in other departments and disciplines which are required of students in this Department, the interdisciplinary character of this work is shown in a particularly significant way by the clinical services programs which are carried on through cooperative arrangements between this Department and other facilities.

THE IOWA PROGRAM AND DENTISTRY

In 1968 cooperation between the Iowa Program and the College of Dentistry, for example, was entering a new phase, in which it is planned that dentists will take training in speech science, and speech pathology and audiology Ph.D.s will take training in certain areas of dentistry. Beginnings of this cooperation, which was part of the pioneering enterprise in the beginning of the Program itself, can be documented as far back as 1932-33 when Lloyd N. Fymbo, later a practicing dentist in Sergeant Bluff, undertook a study of the relation of malocclusion to articulatory defects. His 1933 M.S. thesis, filed in the College of Dentistry [later Health Sciences] Library, is a report of that study.

As with all graduate degrees in the early years of the Program, the degree was in something other than speech pathology. Fymbo's was in the Department of Orthodontia of the College of Dentistry. In his preface to the study he acknowledged the help of Dr. J. Elon Rose and Dr. L. Bodine Higley of Orthodontia, and of Lee Travis, Harry Barnes, and Bessie Rasmus of Speech. Except for Dr. Rose, all of these people figured prominently in the Iowa Program during the Travis era.

Ernest Hixon did his research for the M.S. degree in orthodontics under Curtis. Hixon then became head of the Department and provided active leadership in bringing the two programs together. Spriestersbach served on a number of the master's thesis committees in orthodontics and directed two theses, that of Eldon Bills in 1961, and that of Lawrence D. Engmann in 1962.

During the fifties, in the Speech Pathology research program headed by Spriestersbach, cooperation with the College of Dentistry was renewed. It continued in the Curtis period under Morris. The work dealt primarily with the problems of individuals with cleft lip and palate. Coursework on such problems was included in the College of Dentistry curriculum, with a member of the faculty of the Department of Speech Pathology and Audiology in charge.

ASHA NOTABLES

By 1968, the closing year of the Curtis period, the roster of Fellows of the American Speech and Hearing Association carried the names of sixteen past and present members of the Iowa Speech Pathology and Audiology faculty and one extraordinarily staunch friend of the Iowa Program. The sixteen are: Spencer Brown, Curtis, Darley, Fairbanks, Hardy, Johnson, Keaster, Melrose, Moll, Morris, Schubert, Sherman, Small, Spriestersbach, Travis, and Williams. The friend is Dr. Lierle, former head and now emeritus, Department of Otolaryngology and Maxillofacial Surgery, pioneer in audiology, and long-time contributor to that profession and to the work in that area at Iowa in his own Department and in the Iowa Program.

During the period six people who had earned a Ph.D. at Iowa in the pioneer days of the Program were voted Honors of the Association: Fairbanks in 1955, Powers and Van Riper in 1956, Steer in 1958, Bryngelson in 1963, and Koepp-Baker in 1965. (Five other Iowa pioneers were voted Honors awards after the end of the period: Curtis, Darley, Reger, and Spriestersbach in 1969, and Sherman in 1972.)

ASHA EXECUTIVE COUNCIL

Iowa faculty people on the ASHA Executive Council in the period were: Curtis, 1955; Darley, 1956; Darley, 1957; Johnson, 1959; Johnson and Spriestersbach, 1960; Curtis, Johnson, Spriestersbach, and Williams, 1961; Curtis, Johnson, and Spriestersbach, 1962; Curtis and Spriestersbach, 1963; Spriestersbach and Williams, 1964, 1965, 1966; Williams, 1967.

In every year of the thirteen-year period, individuals with advanced degrees from Iowa who were not on the Iowa faculty were also members of the Executive Council. In the order of the beginning year of their terms they were: Margaret Hall Powers, Stanley Ainsworth, Ernest Henrikson, Ruth B. Irwin, Hayes Newby, Wilbert Pronovost, Jack Bangs, Oliver Bloodstein, Earl Schubert, John Black, George Wischner, and William Tiffany. (Schubert was no longer on the Iowa faculty at the time of his election to the Council; Darley served a second term on the Council, 1964-67, when he too was no longer on the Iowa faculty.)

PUBLICATIONS

Books. In the chronology of their copyrights, the books edited and/or authored by the faculty in this period were: *Your Most Enchanted Listener,* by

Johnson (Harper & Row, 1956; in paperback as *Verbal Man, the Enchantment of Words,* Collier, Macmillan, 1966); the revised edition of *Speech Handicapped School Children,* edited by Johnson, written by him and Curtis of the present faculty, and by Spencer Brown, Clarence Edney, and Jacqueline Keaster of the earlier faculty (Harper & Row, 1956); *The Onset of Stuttering,* edited by Johnson, written by him and his associates, including four from the faculty: Darley, W. Prather, Sherman, and Williams (University of Minnesota, 1959); *Stuttering and What You Can Do About It,* by Johnson (University of Minnesota, 1961; in paperback, Dolphin, Doubleday, 1962; in paperback, Interstate Printers and Publishers, 1967); *Diagnostic Methods in Speech Pathology,* by Johnson, Darley, and Spriestersbach, a revision of their 1952 *Diagnostic Manual in Speech Correction* (Harper & Row, 1963; translated into Japanese by Sumiko Sasanuma and associates for distribution in Japan by Harper & Row); *Speech Handicapped School Children,* third edition, edited by Johnson and Dorothy Moeller (Harper & Row, 1967); *Because I Stutter,* by Johnson, microfilmed or xerographed copies of the 1932 publication (University Microfilm Library Services, Ann Arbor, 1967); *Cleft Palate and Communication,* edited by Spriestersbach and Sherman, with chapters by several authors including Curtis, Moll, Morris, Prather, and Spriestersbach of, or formerly of, the faculty (Academic Press, 1968).

Booklets. Booklets of the period include: Johnson's "Toward Understanding Stuttering," in the parent series of the National Society for Crippled Children and Adults, 1958; "Hearing Rehabilitation," by Prather, in a series of booklets distributed by the Department of Otolaryngology and Maxillofacial Surgery, 1962; and contributions by Johnson and Williams in booklets of the Speech Foundation of America.

Books in Process. In 1968 two books were in process, Hardy writing one, Spriestersbach the other.

Hardy's book will be called *Speech Production Problems of Children With Cerebral Palsy.* He will include results of his decade of research on children with cerebral palsy, and will emphasize suggestions for the clinical management of speech disorders that are associated with conditions of cerebral palsy.

Spriestersbach's work is the first volume of a two-volume publication based on his research of psychosocial problems related to cleft lip and/or palate. In this volume he is presenting analyses and evaluations of data collected in this extended study, described earlier in this chapter. The second volume is completed; it might be described as one long table, including as it does the accumulated interview data which are perhaps the most intensive and extensive in the field today. Nothing had been attempted in such an organized fashion before this study and nothing of this magnitude has been done since.

Chapters. Although Lee Travis' *Handbook of Speech Pathology* (Appleton-Century-Crofts, 1957) was by no means an Iowa production, twelve of its twenty-eight chapter authors have graduate degrees from the Iowa Program, or had been Iowa faculty members, or both. They are: Stanley Ainsworth, Giles Gray, Theodore Hanley, Johnson, Koepp-Baker, Robert Milisen, Powers, Clarence Simon, Mack Steer, Travis, Charles Van Riper, and Robert West.

Iowa faculty members contributed chapters to several other books. They were also represented every year of the period through 1966 in the *Journal of Speech and Hearing Disorders,* and in every year of the period, except 1964, in the *Journal of Speech and Hearing Research* beginning with its first issue in 1958.

EDITORIAL SERVICES

Iowans and former Iowans served in editorial capacities on several of the scholarly journals in the field during the Curtis period.

Editorial Services, ACPA: Morris had been editor of the *Cleft Palate Journal* of the American Cleft Palate Association since 1962 (it was called *Cleft Palate Bulletin* the first year).

Editorial Services, Monographs. Darley was editor of the *Journal of Speech and Hearing Disorders Monograph Supplements* of the American Speech and Hearing Association 1960-1962. *Monograph No. 5,* 1959, "Research Needs in Speech Pathology," was sponsored by the ASHA research committee of which Johnson was a member. *Monograph No. 6,* 1960, "The Problem of Stuttering in Certain North American Indian Societies," and *No. 7,* 1961, "Studies of Speech Disfluency and Rate of Stutterers and Nonstutterers," were edited by Johnson and written by graduate students in the Department. He was also an author in *No. 7. Monograph No. 8,* 1961, "Public School Speech and Hearing Services," another issue sponsored by the ASHA research committee with Johnson a member, was edited by Darley.

When the Association voted in 1963 to discontinue the *JSHD Monograph Supplements* series in favor of two new publications, *ASHA Monographs* and *ASHA Reports,* Maryjane Rees (Iowa Ph.D. 1954) became editor of the former until 1968, when Gerald Siegel (Iowa Ph.D. 1957) succeeded her. Darley became editor of *ASHA Reports* in 1968.

The first issue of *Reports,* April 1965, carried papers given by Spriestersbach, Moll, and Hardy at a 1963 conference sponsored by ASHA and the National Institute of Dental Research. The second issue, September 1967, covered a conference on hearing aid evaluation supported by a Children's Bureau grant. Melrose served on a research subcommittee and chaired two panel discussions. Lilly was a panelist.

Editorial Services, JSHR. When ASHA established the *Journal of Speech and Hearing Research* in 1957, Sherman was named its first editor. She served until March 1963, when she was succeeded by James Jerger.

In the beginning she named Darley as a consultant on editorial problems and policies; in 1960, Small, as an associate editor, and Moll and Martin Young (Iowa Ph.D. 1960) as assistant editors; and in 1962, Moll, as an associate editor. Assistants to the editor were Jean Kern, 1957-58, and Dorothy Moeller, 1958-63. Under Jerger's editorship, Williams became an editorial consultant and later four others from the Iowa faculty were named associate editors: Lilly, Melrose, Moll, and Small.

Editorial Services, JSHD. Associate editors on the staff of the *Journal of Speech and Hearing Disorders* during the Curtis period included Sherman in statistics, Darley in organic speech disorders, and Williams in stuttering. In 1968 Melrose became an editorial consultant, as did three former Iowa faculty people, Darley, Jordan, and Schubert.

Editorial Services, JSHD plus JSHR. Members of the Iowa faculty or persons with an Iowa Ph.D. have served half of the total number of editor-years required to produce ASHA's *Journal of Speech and Hearing Disorders* and *Journal of Speech and Hearing Research* from the beginning in 1936 up to 1968, that is, twenty-one years out of forty-two.

Editorial Services, dsh Abstracts. As Chairman (1959-1962) of the ASHA Publications Board, Johnson joined others from the Association and from Gallaudet College as a founding member of a service unit called Deafness Speech and Hearing Publications (see Article X, section 15, ASHA by-laws) which publishes a quarterly journal called *dsh Abstracts.* Spriestersbach was also a member of the *dsh* board, one year as chairman. The first issue of *dsh Abstracts* appeared in October 1960. Function of the publication is, as the name suggests, to present abstracts of studies on deafness, speech, and hearing (see *Asha 2:8,* August 1960, 246-249).

Editorial Services, Asha. Five present and former members of the Iowa faculty have served on the staff of *Asha* since this news publication of ASHA first appeared the fall of 1959. Schubert in 1959-60, Spriestersbach and Schubert in 1961, and Williams in 1962 and 1963, have all been associate editors. Morris, Williams, and Darley are on its publication board.

DEDICATION WEEK

Dedication week for the Wendell Johnson Speech and Hearing Center, June 11-15, 1968, an event of significance in the closing months of the Curtis period, was in part a homecoming because it brought back scores of people who had had a connection with the Iowa Program at some point down through the years. For the most part, however, the focus was on the future. The conference looked at major issues in doctoral training in speech pathology. The address was on specific needs in the broad area of human communication. The tribute to Wendell Johnson was a tribute not only to the man, a scholar, and a friend, but also to his ideas, which have "challenged us to revise our perspectives and conceptions." During the week Curtis gave voice on several occasions not to history but to the "new opportunities presented by the new facilities."

Lewis (5) found himself pleased to remember that years ago he had favored "Speech and Hearing Science or Speech and Hearing Research or something like that" as the name of the new department. That was during the weekly sack-lunch discussions of the faculty in the old Gables, during the time of the Council, when Johnson was chairman and when Lewis was teaching courses in the Program. Lewis's idea had not been accepted. There was the feeling that the title might be confusing, since Otolaryngology was concerned with speech and hearing science and had a research program in that area. Now, however, Lewis saw at least part of that early-day suggestion put to use in the name of the new building: The Wendell Johnson Speech and Hearing Center.

THE DEDICATION CONFERENCE

The seventy-five participants in the dedication-week conference represented more than fifty of the major doctoral training programs in the United States, as well as four federal granting agencies sponsoring traineeships and research programs in speech pathology and audiology. In the June Department Newsletter the sessions were described as "stimulating, even heated," and the point was made that though perhaps few issues were resolved, "the free and open discussions sharply brought them into focus and will no doubt have a very dramatic impact in many subtle ways on the future of our field."

Curtis and Spriestersbach opened the conference. Strother, of the University of Washington, gave the keynote address, looking at the sometimes conflicting claims of social responsibility and professional status in the face of today's increased and increasing demands for speech and hearing services. Two other former faculty members, Schubert of Stanford (Iowa Ph.D. 1948), and Darley of the Mayo Clinic, appeared on the program. So did John Black of Ohio State (Iowa Ph.D. 1935). Among those in the audience who had taught at Iowa in an earlier day were Brown of Yale and Darien, Connecticut (Iowa Ph.D. 1937), who had been on the faculty from 1947 to 1949; Powers, Director of the Bureau of Physically Handicapped Children for the Chicago public school system (Iowa Ph.D. 1938), who had been a teaching assistant to Travis while she was a doctoral candidate; Keaster of Childrens Hospital, Los Angeles, who had held a joint appointment in Otolaryngology and the Department from 1945 to 1953; Reger of Otolaryngology at Iowa (Iowa Ph.D. 1933) who had been "loaned" to the Program, the Council, and the Department for varying portions of his time from 1931 to that day; Jeanne Smith of Otolaryngology, who had been full-time in that Department since 1953, but who had always been a part of Speech Pathology and Audiology; and Bessie Rasmus Petersen of Iowa City (Iowa M.A. 1930), who had been one of the earliest clinicians working with Samuel Orton and Travis during the decade that began with her B.A. in 1926.

Current faculty on the conference program included Curtis, Hardy, Lilly, Melrose, Moll, Morris, Small, Spriestersbach, and Williams. Prather and Evan Jordan, on the faculty earlier in the Curtis period, were among the conference participants.

THE ALUMNI BANQUET

At the alumni banquet, with Melrose as master of ceremonies, the program turned mellow as Koepp-Baker of Southern Illinois, Steer of Purdue (each of whom received an Iowa Ph.D. in 1938), Darley of Mayo's, and Reger of Iowa told "how it really was."

DEDICATION CEREMONIES

Dedication ceremonies on June 15, held outdoors in the sunshine near the new Center, brought to a close and a climax the week's events. Curtis presided. Johnson's longtime friend, Dr. Richard L. Masland, from 1959 to 1968 Director of the National Institute of Neurological Diseases and Blindness (now the National Institute of Neurological Diseases and Strokes), spoke on "Human Communication." President Stanley Redeker of the Board of Regents formally presented the Center to the University, and President Howard R. Bowen of the University formally accepted it. The Johnson family's close friend, Reverend Evans Worthley, eighty-six, for many years retired and then living near Sterling, Colorado, had driven from there with Mrs. Worthley to be present and to give the invocation and closing prayer.

The tribute to Johnson was by another close friend, Dean Spriestersbach, who chose to use Johnson's own words, explaining "I am unable to take the measure of the man Wendell Johnson and therefore I will not attempt it. Rather, I shall share with you some of the things that he has written and said, for we pay tribute to him today and we memorialize this building to him because of his ideas. They will serve as the time-binders between him and us and our successors." He proceeded then to read a score of these ideas as Johnson himself had stated them.

At the end Mrs. Johnson, escorted to the platform by her son Nicholas and with her daughter Katie and others of the family looking on, unveiled a plaque which is now mounted in the entrance area of the Center. On it were these words, written by Johnson for a talk to a group of students December 10, 1954:

> To be curious, to investigate,
> To think, to learn,
> To become as fully aware as possible
>   of one's self and of one's world,
> To evaluate tradition
>   with the calm and appreciative honesty
>   that one employs in evaluating
>   new knowledge and points of view,
> And so
> To leave the world a bit more favorable
>   to the full flowering
>   of each individual in it—
> These things, to me, are important.
>   —Wendell Johnson

It was with the reading of these words that Spriestersbach concluded his tribute. And it was then with Reverend Worthley's prayer and the Redeker-to-Bowen presentation that the dedication ceremony ended. The Iowa Program in Speech Pathology and Audiology was now officially at home in the Wendell Johnson Speech and Hearing Center, a block and a half, and forty-four productive and amazing years, removed from Travis' little laboratory in the basement rooms in the Psychopathic Hospital just over the hill, where it all had started.

END AND BEGINNING

The Curtis period ended three months after the dedication when Curtis, having resigned administrative duties to give full time to teaching and research, was succeeded by Kenneth Moll, fifth head of the Program, second head of the Department. At about the same time, Curtis and his colleagues realized a major achievement, perhaps the capstone of the period, in the revision of curricula which was announced in University catalogue No. 1968 for the 1968-1969 academic year. This was the final and most thoroughgoing of the three accomplished in the period. It was produced by the entire faculty working through a revision committee whose members were Anderson, Curtis, and Sherman, with Hardy as chairman. Much of the catalogue copy is taken from this committee's report. The revision has been called the current expression of an educational philosophy as old as the Program and supported with unusual vigor throughout this period. Resources within the faculty to implement the revised curricula are suggested by the range of areas covered by research and course content: acoustics, anatomy and physiology of speech and auditory processes, articulation disorders, audiometry, aural rehabilitation, cleft palate, clinical procedures, development of speech and language, hearing science, neural processes and neuropathologies of speech and language, pathologies of audition, psychoacoustics, psycholinguistics, speech science, stuttering, and voice disorders.

EPILOGUE: THE NEXT DECADE

And so, in the fall of 1968, at the beginning of the Moll period, with the new building and the new curricula, what lies ahead for the Department? That question was given at least a partial answer by Curtis and his faculty in these general projections for the 1968-1978 decade, made in their December 1967 Analysis of Program and Recommendations to Dean Stuit:

It is assumed that the graduate enrollment in the Department will increase by about 50 per cent. In part this assumption is governed by what we think constitutes the number of students who can be accommodated in the program without sacrificing the quality of their training. In the clinical training phase . . . certain natural limits . . . are set by the size of the clinical population that is likely to be available. . . . Other phases of the program, e.g., the research program and the graduate training in speech and hearing sciences, do not have this type of natural limitation.

It is further assumed that the number of graduate students for whom the master's degree is the terminal objective will level off in the near future and will increase very little thereafter. This assumption is based on the fact that the number of universities offering master's degrees in this field has increased markedly in recent years. If most of these programs survive and develop, the population of graduate students at the pre-master's degree level will necessarily be more widely distributed that heretofore.

It is assumed also that the number of doctoral candidates enrolled at the University will continue to increase and that, in the future, doctoral students will become a considerably larger proportion of our total graduate student population than is presently the case. This projection is based on the assumptions . . . that there will continue to be a high demand for persons trained at the doctoral level, that some students who earn master's degrees at institutions that do not offer doctoral level work will transfer to Iowa for the latter part of their graduate study, and that a greater portion of students who begin their graduate study in this Department will continue through to the doctorate.

It is assumed that in the future we will attract an increasing number of postdoctoral students. This seems like a reasonable development, if we can develop the types of research programs that should be possible in our new laboratories. Postdoctoral study is becoming increasingly important, especially for those whose primary interests are in speech and hearing science and our new facilities should provide an attractive environment for such study.

It is projected that the Department's research program will develop and expand at an accelerated pace during the next ten years. This seems reasonable [since] . . . the new laboratories provide for a substantial expansion in the research . . . which will be a necessary accompaniment of an increasing emphasis on doctoral and postdoctoral training [also since] . . . the research program must be extended into some new areas . . . if we are to keep pace with developments in the field [and since] . . . we should be able to compete successfully for a reasonable share of . . . federal funds . . . available to support . . . research programs.

Examples of new areas are the application of computer technology to research in speech and hearing science, and the use of small animal research to investigate problems in auditory neurophysiology and auditory psychophysics.

The speech science area has the greatest immediate needs for new development since . . . there is expected to be a substantial increase in demand throughout the country for individuals trained as teachers and researchers [in view of the] general change in the philosophy of undergraduate education in speech pathology and audiology, an example of which is the . . . revised undergraduate program of this Department. . . . In addition, opportunities for positions in speech and hearing science research in academic, government, and industrial laboratories have been increasing in recent years and there seems to be no reason to suppose that this trend will be reversed.

Then, as if to summarize and look ahead, there are these paragraphs:

As is the case with most departments in a large, multipurpose university, the purpose of the Department of Speech Pathology and Audiology is three-fold and includes teaching, research, and service.

The courses and degree programs of the Department are planned to meet the needs of the students having a wide range of career objectives: college and university teachers and researchers, full-time researchers in government and industrial laboratories, and professional clinicians in hospitals, community clinics, rehabilitation centers, public and special schools, etc. Another appropriate division of students, in relation to career interests and objectives, may be made in terms of their primary interest, whether in speech pathology, audiology, or speech and hearing science.

In contrast to corresponding programs in some universities, the University of Iowa Department of Speech Pathology and Audiology has traditionally provided degree programs for students whose sole objective was teaching and research concerned with the fundamental nature of the normal processes of human communication through speech and hearing. In fact this Department prides itself on the quality of scientific training that it affords to students, and its graduates in speech and hearing science are in demand throughout the country.

Research objectives have included the study of both normal and abnormal processes of human communication and have included studies involving the processes of speech production, the development and nature of language behavior, and the processes of audition. Until recently, limitations of both laboratory facilities and staff have limited the research program in both range and amount since the same laboratories had to serve for teaching and also for thesis research, student projects, and faculty research. Often there was competition for both equipment and space. With the completion of the new Center, the Department has, for the first time, the facilities that are needed to enable it to think in terms of major expansion of its research program. Accordingly, in the next few years a good deal of time and effort will be devoted to this.

Because a very important phase of the teaching program of the Department is concerned with the development of clinicians, a clinical service program which serves as the teaching laboratory for the development of clinical skills is a very necessary adjunct of the Department's facilities. Such a clinical service program is also a primary requisite of that portion of the research program which is concerned with the development of knowledge concerning the nature of speech, hearing, and language disorders and the procedures by means of which they may be detected, described adequately for diagnostic purposes, managed therapeutically, etc.

The University of Iowa service programs for persons with speech, hearing, and language disorders include the University Speech and Hearing Clinic, housed in the Speech and Hearing Center [and many departments and agencies of the University and the community]. Thus a very complex program of diagnostic and therapeutic service is provided. The result is that we are able to provide an exceptional range and amount of clinical experience for students. . . . To make full use of this complex of services requires a very substantial amount of interdisciplinary cooperation cutting across both departmental and college lines. Such extensive cooperation is not achieved without effort and a substantial amount of administrative time and effort is required to keep the service program working with reasonable harmony. To aid in this process the position of Director of Clinical Services was created two years ago. . . . Further formal procedures for facilitating the interdisciplinary cooperation that is so essential include the use of joint appointments and courtesy appointments.

With our excellent new facilities we are now presented with new opportunities. . . . We trust we shall prove equal to the challenge which these facilities present.

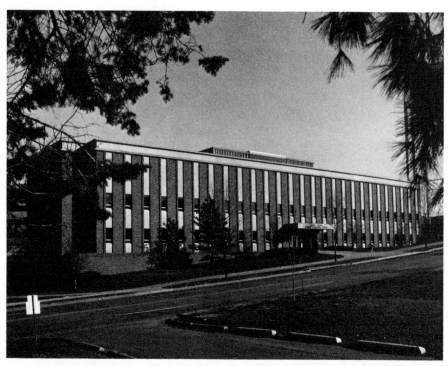

The Wendell Johnson Speech and Hearing Center as it appears today.

REFERENCES

1. Bryng Bryngelson, taped conversation with author, Minneapolis, February 27, 1968.

2. James F. Curtis, taped conversations with author, June 24 and November 22, 1968; January 31, 1969; January 24 and April 6, 1972.

3. Wendell Johnson, "The American Speech and Hearing Foundation," *Asha, 2:* August 1960, 252-5.

4. Wendell Johnson, James F. Curtis, Spencer Brown, Clarence Edney, Jacqueline Keaster, *Speech Handicapped School Children*, third edition, Johnson and Dorothy Moeller, editors (New York: Harper & Row, 1967).

5. Don Lewis, taped conversation with author, Iowa City, October 1, 1969.

6. Dean Lierle, taped conversation with author, Iowa City, September 24, 1969.

7. Jay Melrose, taped replies to questions by author, Iowa City, December 8, 1968.

8. Dorothy Sherman, conversations with author, Iowa City, 1968-1972.

9. Jeanne Kellenberger Smith, conversations and correspondence with author, November 1971, February 22, 1972, and March 1972.

10. D. C. Spriestersbach, taped conversation with author, Iowa City, January 24, 1969, and correspondence, August 6, 1973.

11. Charles Strother, taped conversation with author, Chicago, March 1, 1968, and personal correspondence with author, February 17, 1971, and April 3, 1972.

12. Mildred Templin and Frederic L. Darley, *Templin-Darley Tests of Articulation* (Iowa City: University of Iowa Bureau of Educational Research and Service, Extension Division, 1960).

13. Frank Vance, Division of Special Education, State of Iowa Department of Public Instruction, personal correspondence with author, April 3, 1969.

NOTES

[1] Department Reports are from the files of the Department unless another source is indicated.

[2] National Institute of Neurological Diseases and Blindness, later National Institute of Neurological Diseases and Stroke.

[3] Letters, memos, and other documents cited are from the University archives unless another source is stated. (Department Reports, as noted earlier, are from the files of the Department.)

INDEX

(Proper names, organizations and journals)

Acta Laryngolica, 138
Adams, Lois Hickman, 135
Ainsworth, Stanley, 164, 196, 198
American Academy of Ophthalmology
    and Otolaryngology, 106
American Academy of Speech
    Correction. *See* American Speech
    and Hearing Association
American Association of Cleft Palate
    Prostheses, 133
American Cleft Palate Association, 133,
    164, 171-172, 198
American Hearing Society, 171
American Journal of Physiology, 82
American Otological Society, 66
American Psychological Association,
    109
American Speech and Hearing
    Association (ASHA), 26-27, 39, 41,
    43-44, 52, 58, 81, 93, 97, 108-110,
    114-115, 122, 136, 138, 140,
    146-147, 156, 159, 164-165,
    170-171, 173, 176-177, 180-183,
    184, 185, 188, 196, 198-199
American Speech and Hearing
    Foundation, 165
American Speech Correction
    Association. *See* American Speech
    and Hearing Association
Anderson, Charles, 158, 164, 186, 202
Ansley, Clark, 8
Archives of Neurology and Psychology, 32
Archives of Neurology and Psychiatry, 32,
    82
Archives of Speech, 65, 81, 82
ASHA, see American Speech and
    Hearing Association
    Monographs, 198
    Reports, 198
Atkinson, Chester, 138

Bagchi, Kumar, 48, 71, 97
Baird, Craig, 82
Baldwin, Bird T., 8, 40, 59, 74
Bangs, Jack, 196
Barnes, Harry G., 40, 51, 65, 74, 92, 195
Barrows, Sarah T., 21, 22, 25, 27, 60,
    73-74, 81, 120
Bartell, Bette Rae, *See* Spriestersbach
Bekesy, Georg, 138-139
Bell Telephone Company, 8;
    Laboratories, 69
Bender, Loretta, 31-32
Benton, Arthur, 110, 129, 146
Berg, Lloyd E., 191
Berger, Hans, 68
Berry, Mildred Freburg, 22, 52
Betts, Carl, 158, 164
Bijou, Sidney, 89
Bills, Eldon, 195
Bingham, Dale, 164
Black, John, 49, 69, 100, 119, 136, 137,
    138, 196, 200
Blanton, Margaret, 26 fn
Blanton, Smiley, 26, 26 fn
Blattner, Helene, 66, 73
Bloodstein, Oliver, 149, 196
Bodnar, Andrew, 142
Bolton, B. G., 7
Bontrager, O. R., 188-189
Bordon, Richard, 27 fn
Bowen, Howard R., 183, 185, 186,
    201-202
Boyd, Willard L., 186
Brennan, Thomas, 59, 183
Brown, Frederick, 26 fn
Brown, Judson, 183
Brown, Spencer, 44-45, 55, 71, 90, 94,
    97, 118, 119, 141, 147, 148,
    196-197, 200
Bryngelson, Arminda Mowre, 11, 27, 51

Bryngelson, Bryng, 27-28, 39-42, 44, 49, 52-53, 55, 74, 77. 107, 110, 135, 139, 160, 196

Bunch, C. C., 8-9, 14, 20-21, 46, 59, 64, 66-67, 106-107, 185

Bush, Stephen, 15

Camp, Pauline, 26, 26 fn

Canfield, Norton, 106-107

Carhart, Ray, 106-107, 172

Carr, Josephine, 143, 146

Child Welfare Bulletins, 81

Chotlos, John, 93

Cleft Palate Bulletin. See *Cleft Palate Journal*

Cleft Palate Journal, 198

Cobb, Lois. *See* Kluver

Compton, Arthur, 158

Cordts, Anna D., 21, 22, 81

Council for Medical Education and Hospitals, 172

Council on Speech Pathology and Audiology, 126, 154-155, 160

Cowan, Milton, 30, 48, 53, 74, 81

Craven, Dorothy Drakesmith, 118

Curry, E. Thayer, 148

Curry, F.K.W., 85 fn

Curtis, James F., 39fn, 40, 46, 49, 92, 96, 100-101, 103, 105, 113, 117-119, 125, 127, 129-132, 134-138, 143-146, 147, 148, 149, 154-159, 161-169, 171-174, 176-185, 189, 191, 193, 195-200, 203-205

Daggett, Windsor P., 29

Dahlstron, W. Grant, 146

Darley, Frederic L., 39 fn, 96, 104, 118, 119, 120, 127, 131-134, 141-143. 146, 148, 149, 155, 156, 164, 169, 180, 181, 185, 187, 196, 197, 198, 199, 200, 201

Dassler, Margaret Lee, 95

Davis, Harvey, 122-123, 126, 134

Davis, Mildred, 81

Deafness Speech and Hearing Publications, 199

Dean, L. W., 8, 12, 15, 16, 21-22, 59, 64, 66

Demosthenes Club, The, 92-93, 114, 165

Dolch, John, 138

Dorsey, John, 68

Douglas, Leigh Carroll, 94

Drakesmith, Dorothy, *See* Craven

Dripps, Elaine, 155, 186

Drummond, A. M., 29

dsh Abstracts, 199

Durrell, Don, 32

Edney, Clarence, 148, 197

Egan, James, 47

Elliott, Rep. Carl, 162

Emge, Marie, 155, 186

Engmann, Lawrence D., 195

Eron, Leonard, 183

Estabrook, Eudora, 26 fn

ETC., 106, 170, 188

Fagan, Leo, 45, 74

Fairbanks, Grant, 30, 39-40, 42, 45, 48-49, 70, 72, 74, 81, 88-89, 92, 96-97, 99-105, 117, 119, 120, 142, 147, 148, 154, 160, 181, 183, 196

Falvey, Delta, 187

Farber, I. E., 93

Favors, Aaron, 155, 186

Fisher, Cletus, 158, 164, 186, 191

Fisk, Charlotte, 32

Fladeland, Sina, 26 fn

Fletcher, John, 20, 73, 135

Font, Marion McKenzie, 20, 135

Ford, A. N., 33

Fossler, Harold, 45

Fossum, Ernest, 144

Freund, 33

Froeschels, Emil, 49

Fymbo, Lloyd N., 51, 195

Gallup, George, 43

Gardner, Warren, 50, 51, 79-80

General Semantics Bulletin, 188-189

Giangreco, C. Joseph, 191

Gifford, Mabel, 26 fn

Gilmore, Eugene, 115 fn

Glaspey, Esther, *See* Ogdahl

Glassman, Florence, *See* Saks

Glick, Frank, 54, 122, 183

Goldstein, Max, 26 fn

Gray, Giles, 27, 29, 73-74, 81, 119, 198

Green, Ruth, 26 fn

Gregory, H. H., 85 fn

Gretteman, Theodore J., 109

Griffith, Paul, 19, 68, 70, 72, 137

Grings, William, 95

Guthrie, M. B., 7

Hale, Mark, 122, 183

Hall, G. Stanley, 1-2, 7, 12

Hancher, Virgil M., 109, 115, 115 fn,
117, 118, 183
Hanley, Theodore, 198
Hardy, James C., 156, 158, 164,
169-170, 176, 186, 196-198, 201,
202
Harper, E. E., 93-94
Harshbarger, Clay, 183
Hast, Malcolm, 157-158, 164, 176
Hawk, Sara Stinchfield, 8, 20, 26, 26 fn,
40, 44, 110, 147
Hebenstreit, Marion Brehm, 20, 135
Heltman, H. J., 81
Henrikson, Ernest, 49, 55, 147, 196
Henry, C. E., 48
Herren, Yorke, 45, 68
Herren, Mrs. Yorke, 32
Higley, L. Bodine, 51, 195
Hill Family Foundation, 128, 134, 174
Hiser, Velma Bissell, 144
Hitchcock, Orville, 183
Hixon, Ernest, 195
Hollein, Harry, 163
Horn, Ernest, 22
Horner, George, 125
Houser, Gilbert, 15
Howe, Clifford E., 191
Hull, Catherine J., *See* Van Riper
Hunter, Ted, 33-36, 68, 70, 137
Huston, Paul, 139 fn, 183

Ingram, W. R., 102
Institute of Child Behavior and
Development, 7-8, 25, 40, 59, 74,
90-91, 102, 122, 183
Institute of General Semantics, 113
International Congress on Cleft Palate,
172
International Society for General
Semantics, 106, 110, 113
Iowa Alumni Review, 170
Iowa Child Welfare Research Station.
See Institute of Child Behavior and
Development
Iowa City Press-Citizen, 188
Iowa Committee for the Conservation of
Hearing, 164, 176
Iowa Society for Crippled Children and
Adults, 109, 114, 128, 144
Iowa Speech and Hearing Association,
114, 144-146, 164, 193
Iowa Speech Correction Association. *See*
Iowa Speech and Hearing
Association

Iowa State Services for Crippled
Children, 119, 128, 129, 146, 158,
167, 176, 194
Iowa Studies, 80
Iowa Therapist, The, 143, 146, 193
Irwin, Orvis, 92
Irwin, Ruth B., 196

Jackson, Robert, 109
Jacobsen, Carlyle, 110, 122
Jasper, Herbert, 48
Jensen, Paul, 142, 163
Jerger, James, 199
Jessup, Walter A., 12, 22, 64, 115 fn,
122
Johnson County Society for Crippled
Children and Adults, 142
Johnson, Katy, 201
Johnson, Kenneth, 184
Johnson, Mrs. Wendell, 201
Johnson, Nicholas, 201
Johnson, Wendell, 14, 17, 30, 39-41,
44-45, 47-53, 55, 59, 61-63, 70-78,
80-81, 88-89, 92-98, 99-106, 110,
113-135, 140, 141, 143, 144, 146,
147, 148, 149, 150, 154-156, 159,
162, 163, 165, 168-169, 170, 171,
174, 179-183, 185, 188, 192,
196-199, 201
Jones, Howard, 183
Jones, R. K., 85 fn
Jordan, Evan, 156, 164-165, 176, 187,
199, 201
Jordan, Herbert, 186
Jordan, Linda Smith, 155-156, 186
Journal of Experimental Psychology, 82
Journal of General Psychology, 82
*Journal of Neurology, Neurosurgery, and
Psychiatry,* 85
Journal of Speech and Hearing Research,
85, 156, 180, 192, 198, 199
*Journal of Speech Disorders. See Journal of
Speech and Hearing Disorders*
Journal of Speech and Hearing Disorders,
81, 94, 106, 108, 110, 114-115,
120-121, 134, 136, 147-148, 150,
199;
Monograph Supplements, 148, 198
Journal of Speech and Hearing Research,
180, 192, 197-199

Kay, George, 70, 122
Keaster, Jacqueline, 92, 96, 102-103,
119, 127, 131, 134, 143-144, 148,
157, 196, 197, 200

Kellenberger, Jeanne, *See* Smith
Kelly, George, 45
Kelly, Joseph P., 49
Kenyon, Elmer, 26 fn
Kern, Jean, 199
Klein, Dottie, *See* Ray
Kluver, Lois Cobb, 46, 52
Knabe, Judith Milisen, 155, 186
Knott, John, 44-45, 48, 55, 68, 71, 75-78, 81, 88, 97, 102, 118, 137, 140
Knower, Franklin, 65, 92
Koepp-Baker, Herbert, 39-40, 43, 107, 110, 133, 147, 148, 196, 198, 201
Korzybski, Alfred, 74
Kos, C. M., 164

Lacy, Mabel, 26 fn
Ladd, George Trumbull, 2, 18
Lampe, Dorothy McGlone, 32
Lee, Bernard S., 137
Leutenegger, Ralph R., 134
Lewin, Kurt, 90-91
Lewis, Don, 17, 30, 46-48, 51, 69, 72-74, 93-96, 100, 104-105, 118, 119, 120, 124, 136, 157, 200
Lichty, William, 95
Lierle, Dean, 46, 49-50, 59, 66-67, 79, 91, 99, 107-108, 117-118, 120, 122, 126-127, 129, 163-164, 168, 183, 196
Lilly, David, 158, 165, 199, 201
Lindeman, Eric, 55, 90
Lindquist, E. F., 18
Lindsley, D. B., 48
Loehwing, Walter F., 123, 125, 126, 129, 183
Lyday, June F., 31, 32
Lynch, Gladys, 49, 92, 102-104, 117, 119, 132, 154, 159, 161

Mabie, Edward C., 15, 16, 18, 27-31, 42, 59, 65, 74, 82, 90, 96, 98, 103, 123, 125-126, 129, 134, 135, 140, 144, 159-162, 183-184, 192
MacEwen, Ewen, 18, 102
MacLean, George E., 7
Malamud, William, 55, 77, 90
Masland, Richard, 163, 201
Maucker, William, 100
McBride, Mary Margaret, 149
McBroom, Maude, 22, 101
McCabe, Brian, 120, 163-164, 183
McCandless, Boyd, 122, 129, 183
McClintock, J. T., 17, 18
McDermott, Richard, 156

McDowell, Floyd M., 15
McGeoch, John, 88, 91
McGlone, Dorothy, *See* Lampe
McGrath, Earl, 122
Melrose, Jay, 42, 158, 164, 181, 186, 193-194, 196, 199, 201
Mental Hygiene, 31
Merry, Glenn T., 9-11, 14, 18, 20-22, 29-30, 48, 59, 73, 74, 119, 160
Metfessel, Milton, 18, 25, 27, 29, 30, 36, 45, 48, 74, 81-82, 119, 121-122, 124, 154
Milisen, Robert, 49, 51, 71, 97-98, 148, 198
Miller, Wilbur, 183
Mills, Alice, 22, 27, 120
Moeller, Barbara, 186, 197
Moeller, Dorothy, 197, 199
Moll, Kenneth, 155-156, 164, 170, 181, 196, 198, 199, 201, 202, 203
Monroe, Marian, 32, 33
Morley, Alonzo, 49
Morris, Delyte, 39-40, 43, 49, 81, 147, 148
Morris, Hughlett, 156, 164, 168, 170, 181, 186, 196, 197, 199, 201
Moser, Henry, 49
Mowre, Arminda, *See* Bryngelson
Murray, Elwood, 45, 65, 74
Muyskens, J. H., 26
National Association of Teachers of Speech, 11, 21, 26, 30
National Council for Accreditation of Teacher Education, 172
National Commission on Accrediting, 172
National Institute of Dental Research, 163, 170, 173, 180-181, 198
National Institute of Mental Health, 170
National Institute of Neurological Diseases and Blindness. *See* National Institute of Neurological Diseases and Stroke
National Institute of Neurological Diseases and Stroke, 163-164, 170-171, 180-181, 201
National Institutes of Health, 168-169, 181
National Research Council, 23, 25, 29, 32, 37, 93
National Science Foundation, 169
National Society for Crippled Children and Adults, 93, 109, 115, 197

Neelley, James, 156
Newburn, Harry K., 122
Newby, Hayes, 26, 40, 107-108, 196
Newhart, Horace, 107
Newman, Parley, 142
Nichols, Thyrza, 26 fn

Obermann, C. Esco, 51
Ogdahl, Esther Glaspey, 50
Ogura, Joseph, 164
O'Neill, James M., 27-28
Orton, Samuel, 7, 12, 14-19, 22, 31-33,
    45, 55, 59, 61, 81, 118, 183, 201

Packer, Paul, 65, 79
Parker, Charles, 118, 120, 132, 134,
    155, 157, 164, 181
Parker, Jean, 146
Parker, Jessie, 145
Patrick, George Thomas White, 1-2, 12,
    81
Pepler, Della, 32
Persons, Stow, 183
Petersen, Bessie Rasmus, 26, 32, 45-46,
    51, 56, 66, 70-71, 72, 73-74, 120,
    195, 201
Peterson, E. T., 145, 146, 183
Phillips, Chester A., 115 fn
Phillips, Dorothy, 109, 144
Potter, Ada, 32
Powers, Margaret Hall, 39-40, 43,
    54-55, 68, 71, 72-73, 147, 196, 198,
    200
Prather, William, 157, 164, 176, 197,
    201
Prentiss, Henry, 17, 60
Pronovost, Wilbert, 196
Psychological Monographs, 81
Psychological Review, 81, 121
Quarterly Journal of Speech, 21, 29, 82,
    134
Quarterly Journal of Speech Education. See
    Quarterly Journal of Speech
Raimy, Victor, 110
Rasmus, Bessie, *See* Petersen
Rasmussen, Vera Travis, 49
Ray, Dottie Klein, 52
Redeker, Stanley, 201-202
Rees, Maryjane, 142, 198
Reger, Scott, 17-19, 39 fn, 46-47, 48, 50,
    59, 66-68, 72-73, 79, 88, 91, 97,
    101-103, 107, 117, 120, 125, 127,
    131-132, 134, 138-139, 143, 146,
    147, 157, 183, 200, 201

Rembolt, R. R., 109, 122, 126-127, 129
Ricci, Norma Ames, 146
Ritzman, Carl, 139
Robbins, Samuel, 26 fn
Roe, Vivian, 51
Rose, J. Elon, 51, 195
Rosenbaum, Robert Lee, 143
Ruch, G. M., 18
Ruckmick, Christian, 81
Russell, G. Oscar, 26, 81, 147

Saks, Florence Glassman, 50
Sasanuma, Sumiko, 165, 197
Scheldrup, E. W., 99, 102
Schenke, Lowell B., 142, 143
Schubert, Earl, 93, 96, 118, 119, 120,
    127, 129, 131-132, 134, 137-138,
    146, 155, 157, 163, 181, 196, 199,
    200
Schubert, Mrs. Earl, 104-105, 141
Schuell, Hildred, 98-100, 141
Science, 36, 37, 60, 82, 121
Scientific Monthly, The, 36
Scripture, E. W., 2-4, 12, 49
Sears, Robert, 90-91, 122
Seashore, Carl Emil, 2-12, 14-20, 22-23,
    25-26, 28-30, 33-34, 36, 39-40,
    42-43, 45-47, 50-53, 58-60, 64-70,
    75, 78-82, 90-91, 96, 99, 101, 106,
    110, 115-116, 120-123, 129, 134,
    154, 159, 165, 184, 192
Seibel, Robert, 138
Shackson, Rolland, 49
Shapley, James, 157, 164
Shaw, S. Spencer, 135
Sheehan, Joe, 95
Sherman, Dorothy, 39 fn, 51, 52, 78-79,
    105, 118, 119, 120, 127, 131, 132,
    134, 136-137, 144, 146, 148, 155,
    156, 170, 176, 179, 180, 186, 193,
    196, 197-199, 202
Shover, Jayne, 50, 54
Shriner, Ralph, 183
Siegel, Gerald, 198
Sies, Luther, 176
Simon, Clarence, 18, 40, 44, 81, 106,
    110, 147, 198
Simonson, Josephine, 144
Small, Arnold, 47, 157-158, 169, 179,
    196, 199, 201
Small, Arnold, Sr., 47
Smith, Jeanne Kellenberger, 50, 74,
    104, 119, 157, 164, 176, 181, 201
Smith, Marceline, 144

Snidecor, John, 47
Solomon, Meyer, 26
Speech Correction Foundation, 114-115
Speech Correction Fund, 93, 113, 165
Speech Foundation of America, 197
Spence, Kenneth, 91, 99, 123, 126, 183
Spiker, Charles, 183
Spriestersbach, Bette Rae Bartell, 87, 144, 155, 186
Spriestersbach, Duane C., 39 fn, 40, 92, 96, 118, 120, 126-127, 129, 131-134, 140, 146, 148, 149-151, 155-156, 160-161, 163-164, 168-172, 175, 179-184, 188, 196-202
Stansell, Barbara, 142
State Department of Public Instruction, 193-194;
Division of Special Education, 176
Steer, Mack D., 39-40, 42-43, 71, 97, 100, 134, 147, 196, 198, 201
Steindler, Arthur, 35, 108
Stewart, George W., 9, 17, 157, 159, 160-161
Stoddard, George, 14 fn, 59, 88, 91, 93, 134, 148, 184, 192
Stoelting, 4, 5
Strother, Charles, 49-50, 54, 86-91, 97-101, 103-106, 108-110, 113-114, 117, 119, 125, 126, 144, 147, 154, 159-160, 181, 183, 185, 192, 200
Stroud, James, 129, 146, 191
Stuit, Dewey, 92, 96, 100-101, 122-123, 126, 129, 154, 162, 166, 186, 203
Switzer, Mary, 163, 183

Taylor, Eleanor K., 122
Taylor, Jane, 26 fn
Teager, Florence E., 41
Templin, Mildred, 170
Thomas, C. K., 26 fn
Thorndike, E. L., 23
Tiffany, William, 151, 196
Tiffin, Joseph, 30, 45, 47-48, 65, 69-70, 72, 74, 81, 82, 92, 121, 124, 154
Tonndorf, Juergen, 157
Torrance, Peggy, 32
Travis, Lee Edward, 2, 10, 14-20, 22-40, 42, 44-46, 48-52, 55-62, 64, 66-69, 71-77, 79, 81-83, 86-88, 96, 101-102, 110, 113, 118, 121, 126, 133-135, 137, 139, 139 fn, 147, 154, 157, 159-160, 183, 185, 191, 192, 196, 198, 201, 202
Travis, Vera, *See* Rasmussen
Trotter, William, 105

Tuthill, Curtis, 49
Tuthill, Dorothy Davis, 49, 54
Tuttle, W. W., 81
United States Children's Bureau, 128, 176
United States Civil Service Commission, 164-165
United States House of Representatives, Committee on Education and Labor, 163, 171
United States Office of Education, 163, 171, 172
United States Public Health Service, 109
United States Veterans Administration, 109, 171
University of Iowa Service Bulletin, 31, 60
University of Iowa Studies in Psychology, 81
Van Demark, Ann, 186
Van Demark, Duane, 156, 165, 186
Van Epps, E. F., 7, 18
Van Riper, Catherine J. Hull, 76
Van Riper, Charles, 39-40, 41-42, 44, 53-54, 61-62, 71, 75-76, 81, 83, 97-98, 139, 140, 196, 198
Vasey, Wayne, 122, 129
Vocational Rehabilitation Administration, 163, 169, 171
Voots, Richard, 138, 157
Walker, Betty, 36, 71-72
Ward, Lavilla, 26 fn
Weaver, John, 183
Weaver, Ross, 144
Wellman, Beth, 81, 122
Wendell Johnson Speech and Hearing Center, 154, 187, 191, 199-202
Wernick, Joel, 158
West, Robert, 26, 26 fn, 28, 49, 198
Westlake, Harold, 107
Whitebook, Jan, 186
Williams, Dean E., 118, 155-156, 158, 159, 163, 169, 176, 179, 181, 186, 187, 196, 197, 199, 201
Williams, Dorothy, 146
Williams, Mabel Claire, 10
Wischner, George, 136, 148, 196
Woods, Andrew, 50, 59, 70, 183
Woolbert, Charles, 29, 49, 74, 160
Worthley, Evans, 201-202
Worthley, Mrs. Evans, 201
Wundt, Wilhelm, 1-2, 12
Young, Martin, 199
Zimmerman, Jane Dorsey, 26 fn
Zwaardemaker, Hendrik, 37

SUBJECT INDEX

Acoustics
    and psychology of music, 47
    beginning of as science, 48
    in coursework, 202
    methodology borrowed, 30
    phased out, 157
    see also Psychoacoustics
Accreditation and American Speech
    and Hearing Association, 172
action current research, 33
action potential
    recording equipment, 33, 35
    stuttering and, 49
American Speech and Hearing
    Association (ASHA)
    and accreditation, housing in Curtis
        term, 171-172
    designing of national headquarters
        in Spriestersbach term, 184
    Honors awards to Iowans, 18, 39,
        40, 110, 122, 147, 196
    Iowa Fellows of, 196
    Iowa presidents of, 40
    organized at Travis home, 26-27
    Seashore Honors text from, 122
Amplifiers
    early, 19
    made for others, 68
Aphasia
    and Darley, 120, 180
    and Schuell, 98
    sophistication in work with, 89
    Travis' interest in, 61
Art, psychologist/psychology of, 14
Articulation
    disorders of, 203
    early clinical work in, 71
    physiology of, 181
    problems found in, 66
    research in, 169
    see also Voice and articulation

Audiology
    and Bunch degree, 21
    as emerging discipline, 86
    as new discipline, 106-108
    audiometric, 21, 66
    before word coined, 67
    clinical, 157, 158
    in Curtis period, 157-158
    in Johnson period, 120
    neurophysiology and, 158
    physiological processes in, 203
    psychoacoustics in, 157, 158
    rehabilitative, 157-158
    testing procedures in, 158
Audiometer
    Bekesy's and Reger's, 138-139
    Iowa Pitch Range, 8, 67
    Seashore's, 4-5
    Stoelting marketing of Seashore's,
        4-5
Audiometry
    early courses in, 72
    in Department, 203
    procedures standardized, 59
    pure-tone, 21
    Reger manual on, 139
    slow start in, 3
Audiospectrometer, 138
Auditory stimulation method, 21, 27, 66

B.A., terminal, move from, 136
Backward play, Sherman, 136-137
Brain
    damage, 159
    dissection of, 2
    electrodes in, 61
    models of, 2
    waves and stuttering, 94
    waves recorded by Travis, 64, 68
    waves, recording of and Travis study
        abroad, 37
    see also Dominance theory

Boulder conference and clinical psychology, 109-110

Catalogue listing
see Curriculum
Cerebral dominance theory
see Dominance theory
Cerebral palsy
little done with, 89
research, Hospital School, 156, 180
speech, breathing, and, 169
Certification
basic clinical, 177
campaign for in Iowa schools, 144-146
requirements revised for, 193
Charts and Patrick laboratory, 2
Chief and Duke of Airedale, 52
Child development, 7-8, 90, 92, 110
Psychology, Iowa Program, and, 6
see also (in preceding index) Iowa Child Welfare Research Station, Institute of Child Behavior and Development
McCandless, Sears, Seashore, Stoddard, Wellman
Cineradiography, 169, 180
Cleft lip and palate
first use of obturators, 89
Koepp-Baker's work with, 43
program in, 168, 203
project with Otolaryngology, 155-156, 157
research into, 169, 180
Spriestersbach's work with, 13, 195-196
see also (in preceding index) Lierle, Reger
Climate
and people, 39-56
of beginnings, 1, 2, 4-5
of Curtis period, 203-205
of Johnson period, 149-151
of Strother period, 87-88, 98-100
of Travis period, 39-56
Clinic
Cleft Lip and Cleft Palate, 168
hearing testing mobile, 79-80
Mental Hygiene mobile, 31-33, 45
outpatient, 7, 88
Psychological, of Mental Pathology, 7

Speech and Hearing Mobile, 50-51
SSCC Mobile, 158, 176
supervisors to faculty status, 185-186
see also Psychological and Speech Clinic, Psychological (Psychology) Clinic, Residential Clinic, Speech Clinic
Clinical services
see Services
Clinical procedures, 203
Clinical supervisors to faculty status, 185-186
Common purpose, 54, 58-59, 87
Communication, 54-55, 66, 72, 189, 205
Computer technology in research, 204
Council on Speech Pathology and Audiology
becomes department, 154, 161-162
created, 126
finally in catalogue, 131
for administrative framework, 127-128
organized, 127
proposals for future of, 128-129
Counseling, early, 105
Course listings, *see* Curriculum
Curriculum
early, 72
for 1922-1930, 73-74
for Psychology, 1924-1925, 25-26
in Curtis period, 155-159, 167-168, 177-178, 189-190, 202-203
in Johnson period, 130-132
in Strother period, 101-102
seminars as, 72-73
Deaf, education for, 191-192
Dean of Graduate College, 5, 184-185
Death of pioneers
Johnson, 182, 188-189
Lynch, 159, 161
Mabie, 159-160
Seashore, 120-122
Stewart, 159, 160-161
Decibel and Seashore's rule of thumb, 5
Dentistry, 51, 195-196
Department of Speech Pathology and Audiology
see Speech Pathology and Audiology, Department of
Department of Psychology
see Psychology, Department of

Department of Otology
(Otolaryngology)
see Otology (Otolaryngology)
Department
Department Reports, Curtis period,
166-170, 172-174, 175-177,
178-179, 181-182, 189-190, 195,
203-205
Depression days, 71-72, 87
Diagnosis and appraisal, 119, 156, 180
Disc recorder, 95
Disorders of speech and hearing
see Speech and hearing disorders
Dominance theory of stuttering, 16, 33,
55, 61, 62, 63

East Hall (photo Facing Page 1)
as new home of Program, 64-65
move out of, 192
space problems in, 124-126,
168-169, 178-179, 182
Travis laboratory moved to, 70
electrical potential, muscles, 33
electroencephalography
and Knott, 44, 88
and national leadership, 48-49, 77
see also Electrophysiology
electrodes in brain, 61
Electromyography, 180
Electrophysiology, 44, 60-61, 70, 88,
118, 157
Faculty
ascendancy of Seashore, 5
early changes in, 59
in Curtis period, 155, 183-184, 186,
187
in Johnson period, 117-120,
122-123
in Strother period, 91-92
of three, 103
Fundamentals course, 11, 12, 22, 40, 60,
64, 65, 66, 92

Gables, the, 126
Galvonometer, 69
General Semantics
and Johnson orientation, 74
and stuttering, 105-106
first university course in, 92
in Curtis period, 155
Murray and, 45
Golden era, 56
Graduate degrees, 49, 190-191

Graduate training, Curtis period
shift, in curriculum revision, 154,
167, 177-178, 181, 203, 204
Grant support
during Curtis period, 174
Iowa work with federal agencies,
162-164
Guinea pig, 62

Handedness, 33, 36, 50, 61-62
Harmonic analysis, 30, 70
Head Start program and Clinical
services, 194
Hearing
disorders of and speech problems,
66-67
neuropathologies of, 203
see also Audiology, Audiometry,
Hearing Testing,
Psychoacoustics, Speech and
Hearing Disorders
Hearing testing
conducted by Bunch, 21
in public schools, 79-80
pioneered by Gardner, 50
pulse-tone technique in, 68
Reger's introduction to, 67-68
standardization of for schools, 107
see also Public Schools, Speech
Correction
Henrici Harmonic Analyzer, 69
Honors awards and Iowans, 18, 39, 40,
110, 122, 147, 196
Honors program, 156
Hospital School and Strother, 108-109
laboratory, 180

Individual and speech, 83
Inhibition, Seashore study of, 3
Instruments
amplifiers made and sold, 68
built by
Freund, 33
Griffith, 68
Hunter, 33-36
Lewis, 47, 69
Reger, 19, 67, 138-139
Seashore, 10-11
Tiffin, 69
built for sidetone project, 138
purchase of, 70
waiting for invention, 3
see also specific instrument

Interdisciplinary approach, 6, 10, 12,
    15-16, 17-18, 28-29, 48, 51, 55, 59,
    60, 65, 89-90, 98-100, 106, 115-116,
    158, 159, 194, 195
Iowa Pitch Range audiometer, 8, 67
Iowa Program in Speech Pathology
    and Bunch, Merry, Travis degrees,
        21
    and Merry courses, 10
    beginnings of, 12
    finally in catalogue, 103
    Fletcher and, 20
    followed by Council, 126, 151, 154,
        161-162
    fundamentals course as resource for,
        11, 12, 22, 40, 60, 64, 65, 66, 92
    in Psychology and Speech, 15
    migrates from Psychology to
        Speech, 91, 127
    needs administrative framework,
        116, 123-124
    overview of, 123
    periods of
        Johnson, 113-126
        Patrick, 1-12
        Seashore, 14-122
        Strother, 86-110
        Travis, 25-37, 39-56, 58-83
    philosophy of, 202
    plea for major in, 123
    recognized as entity, 15
    research-professional model for,
        58-59
    Seashore central 20, 5
    Travis work equated with, 23
    University readiness for, 6
Iowa Psychological Laboratory
    see Psychological Laboratory

Kymograph, 32, 33

Laboratory
    and Iowa Program, 30-31
    and new psychology, 1-3
    Cleft Lip and Cleft Palate, 169
    in Hospital School, 180
    inventory in, 19-20
    Patrick's, 2
    with Mental Hygiene Clinic, 31-33
    see also Instrument building
            Phonetics and Speech
                Laboratory

Phonetics and Voice
    Laboratory
Psychological (Psychology)
    Laboratory
Speech Pathology
    Laboratory
Language
    development of, 158, 180, 203
    of Responsibility, 170-171
    neural processes and pathologies of,
        203
Laryngectomees, 50
Leadership of Iowa Scholars in
        Program, Council, Department of
        Speech Pathology and Audiology
    at national level, 18, 39, 40, 106,
        110, 114-115, 122, 133, 147,
        163-164, 171-172, 181, 183, 184,
        196, 198-199
    at state level, 50, 79, 80, 144, 145,
        146, 163, 172, 193
    in Fellows citations, 196
    in Honors awards, 18, 39, 40, 110,
        122, 147-148, 196
    in pioneering, 1-23, 25-37, 39-56,
        58-83, *passim*
Learning to learn, 53
Linguistics
    and Cowan, 47
    as experimental science, 48
    in Curtis period, 189
Literature, lack of, 72
Little girl's problem, 14, 16

malocclusion and speech, 51
Mashburn appartus, 94
M.A. terminal program, 177, 178, 203
Mecca for graduate students, 39
Medicine, College of, and Iowa
    Program, 7, *passim*
Mental and Moral Science and
    Didactics, 5
Mental health, hygiene
    and hopes for mental hospital, 7
    clinical psychology, University
        Hospitals, 87
    laboratory with Mobile Clinic, 31-33
    Mobile Clinic, 31-33, 45
    Psychology, Iowa Program, and, 6
    see also Psychiatry, Psychopathic
            Hospital
Microphones, 69

Migrant workers and clinical services, 194
Mobile clinics
hearing testing, 79-80
Mental Health and Hygiene, 31-33, 45
Speech and Hearing, 50-51
SSCC, 158, 176
Music
and Reger, 46
and Seashore and speech, 10
cineradiography in research in, 181
psychologist/psychology of, 10, 25, 26, 30, 46

Nasality, 49
Nerve potential, broadcast of, 36
Neuropathology, 156
Neurophysiology, 14-15, 16, 61, 77, 158, 180, 204
Noise, high level, and pilots, 94-95
Norms, establishing, 68

Obturators, 89
Onset studies, 71, 132, 133
Open Letter to Mother of Stuttering Child, 165
Organic speech and hearing disorders
and Curtis period, 156, *passim*
and Johnson period, 119, 120
and Strother, 108-109, 113-114
in Hospital School, 108-109
Koepp-Baker and, 43
little noted early, 71
see also Cleft Lip and Palate, Cerebral Palsy
Orthorater, 45
Orton-Travis dominance theory of stuttering, 16, 33, 55, 61, 62, 63, 75-77
Oscillographic techniques, 30
Oscillator, 69
Oscilloscope, 35, 69
Otolaryngology
see Otology
Otolaryngology, Department of
see Otology (Otlaryngology), Department of
Otology (otolaryngology)
as parent of audiology, 107-108
psychologist/psychology of, 9, 46, 106

Otology (Otolaryngology), Department of
and cleft palate program, 155-156, 157
and Psychology, 8-9, 66-67
with Speech, 90, 91
and Speech Clinic committee, 12
cooperates with Program, 5, 9, *passim*
Dean-Bunch program revitalized in, 64, 67
Lierle continues Reger loan from, 117
Program leans less heavily on, 137
Program, Psychology, and, 6
sponsors Program with others, 116, 117
see also (in preceding index) Dean, Lierle, Reger
Outpatient clinics
for Iowa Program, 119
for young mental patients, 7
in Strother period, 88

Philosophy, Seashore as professor of, 2
'Phonelescope, 18, 27, 34
Phonetics
and Barrows, 21, 27
Curtis and, 119
in coursework, 72, 73
in early clinic, 23
in laboratory, 30, 48
physiological and acoustical, 189
Psychology and Speech work in, 65
Phonetics and Speech Laboratory
in 1951 catalogue, 130
listed as major curriculum unit, 135
research program in, 180
space problems of, 125-126
see also Services, Speech Pathology and Audiology Laboratory, Speech Science
Phonetics and Voice Laboratory, 10
Phonology and Voice Laboratory, 10
Phonophotostrobograph, 30
Piano-camera, 69
Pitch, 11, 169
Press relations, Seashore, Travis, 36-37
Principles of speech
see fundamentals course
Problems
little girl's, 14, 16

see also cerebral palsy
cleft lip and palate
hearing
organic speech and hearing
disorders
space
speech and hearing
disorders
Program in Speech Pathology and
Audiology
see Iowa Program in Speech
Pathology and Audiology
Projections, expectations, to 1978,
203-205
Psychiatry
and psychology, 3, 7, 14, 16, 23, 53
psychologist/psychology of, 14
see also Psychology
Psychology, Department of
Psychiatry, Department of
and clinical psychology, 3
and mobile clinic, laboratory, 31-33
and Otology and Psychology, 66
and Program in Strother period, 90
and Psychology and little girl's
problem, 14, 16
and Psychology in Travis period,
25-83
and Psychology in Travis laboratory,
30-31, 32, 33-36
welcomes students from Program,
59
see also (in preceding index)
Huston, Lindeman, Malamud,
Orton, Woods
Psychoacoustics, 5, 46-47, 157, 158, 169,
189, 203
Psycholinguistics, 159-160, 189, 203
Psychological and Speech Clinic
becomes two, 117
before its day, 46
confusing titles of, 70-71
moved to East Hall, 70-71
new emphasis on, 88
separate listings of, 74
Strother director of, 86
Travis director of, 58-59, 60
Psychological (Psychology) Clinic
and Strother, 88
as Seashore innovation, 7
confusion of names of, 59-60
procedures revised in, 89

separated from Speech, 74
separated from Speech Clinic, 117
Travis as director of, 23
Psychological Clinic of Mental
Pathology, 7
Psychological (Psychology) Laboratory
as Seashore's workshop, 4
in Psychopathic Hospital, 58
Patrick in world's and USA's first, 1
listed in catalogue since 1890, 2
Patrick's one of earliest, 2
Seashore director of, 2
Speech gets use of, 30
Strother director of, 88
to East Hall, 64-65
Travis director of, 70
Travis, Metfessel, Reger, Simon in,
18-20
Psychological testing, 32, 50
Psychologist/psychology
of art, 14
of music, 10, 25, 46, 47
of otology, 9, 46, 66, 106
of psychiatry, 14, 66
of speech, 14, 25
Psychology
abnormal, 7
and psychiatry, 3, 14, 16, 23, 53
and speech, 3, 58
and University Diagram, 28-29
applied, two views, 6
clinical, 3, 7, 25, 55, 73, 86, 87,
109-110
creative approach to, 3
industrial and Tiffin, 45
no applied in 1895, 3
of speech, 3
sensory, 157
the "new," 1, 2-3, 28
Psychology, Department of
and conference, ASHA organized,
26
and major department allies, 16-18
and Research Station, 90
and Otology, 8-9
and Psychiatry and little girl's
problem, 14, 16
and Psychiatry and Travis
laboratory, 30-31, 70
and school hearing testing, 79-80
and Speech and Otolaryngology, 91
and Speech Clinic budget, 70

and Speech Clinic committee, 12
cross listing with Speech, 73-74,
    102-103, 130-131
Iowa Program centered in, 15
McGeoch as head, 88
position in University (diagram),
    28-29
Program degrees in, 123
Program migrating from, 90
separates from Philosophy,
    Seashore as head, 5
Spence as head, 91
sponsor of Program, with others,
    116, 117
takes Psychology half of Psychology
    and Speech Clinic, 117, with
    Philosophy, 5
see also Curriculum
(in preceding index) McGeoch,
    Seashore, Spence, Stoddard
Psychometrics, 99
Psychopathic Hospital(s)
and clinical psychology, 3
and Strother, 87, 108
and Travis laboratory, 30-31, 32,
    33-36, 59, 65, 68, 70
establishment at Iowa, 7
see also Psychiatry, Department of
Psychophysics, 204
Psychophysiology, 73
Psychosocial approach, Johnson,
    132-133
Public relations, Seashore and Travis,
    31-37
Public schools
and Iowa leadership for state
    certification, 193
hearing testing in, 78-79
services for, 173, 175
speech correction in, 78-79
speech correction training for, 155,
    166-167
WPA survey of, 93
see also Speech correction
Publications by Iowa scholars
in Curtis period, 156, 180, 188,
    196-198
in Johnson period, 134, 135, 136,
    148
in Strother period, 94, 105, 106, 113
in Travis period, 14, 22, 36, 48, 49,
    64, 75, 80-82, 83

Pulse-tone technique, 68
Radio
early AC tubes, 19
first nerve-current broadcast over,
    36
receiver, new, 35
Rat(s), 27, 36, 61-62
Regional Educational Services
    Administration and Speech Clinic
    services, 194
Rehabilitation, 18, 43, 44, 51, 65, 92
as major thrust in audiology,
    107-108, 203
Research
action current, 33
and computer technology, 204
and little girl, 14-15, 16
and service, 54, 55
basic to clinic, 22-23
basic to Iowa Program, 30-31
challenge in, 53-54
communication and, 54-55
early listing of, 81-82
in articulation, 169
in audiology, 157-158
in new psychology, 1-3
Johnson's cry for help in, 96-98
mark of Travis period, 113
model: research-professional, 58-59
questing, questioning in, 63-64
Seashore's commitment to, 6, 12,
    passim
techniques exhibit of, 170
work for federal support for,
    162-164
Residential Clinic
and summer clinic, 104-105
in Curtis period, 175
in Johnson period, 119, 141-142
reorganization of, 187
social worker and, 187
Respiratory physiology and speech, 156,
    180
Roe-Milisen studies, 51
Scaling
by Lewis, 47, 93-95, 105
by Sherman, 105, 120
in first publication, 136
School of Religion, 5
Schools, public
see Public schools

Seashore Plan, 16-18
Sensory psychology, 157
Seminars as fill-ins, 72-73
Services
    caseload in Clinic, 193-194
    in Curtis period, 156, 167, 173,
        175-177
    reorganization of clinical, 193-194
Sheep's brain, 2
Sidetone project, 137-138
"Some of this I brought," 1
Soundproof room
    anechoic chamber, 135
    dead room, 47
    insulated cage, 68-69
    listening laboratory, 135
    Seashore's thermos bottle, 4, 64
Sound waves
    early analysis of, 69-70
    etched on glass, 69
Space problems
    Gables added to alleviate, 126
    continuing and desperate, 168-169,
        178-179, 182
    in East Hall, 124-126
Speech
    acquisition, 159
    anatomy and physiology of, 202
    and breathing, 169
    and respiratory physiology, 180
    arts, 9-11
    as behavior, Woolbert, 29, 49
    auditory stimulation and, 21-22
    development of, 120, 203
    first scientific approach to, 9, 10, 11
    neural processes and
        neuropathologies of, 203
    psychologist/psychology of, 3, 14,
        25, 26,
    sounds graphed, 11
Speech, Department of
    adds laboratory, 30
    and Psychology, 58
    and Psychology with Otology, 91
    and Speech Clinic, 65
    and Speech Clinic committee, 12
    and speech science, 135-136
    cross listing with Psychology, 73-74,
        102-103, 130-131, 132
    denied Ph.D. program, 29
    fundamentals course in, 11, 12, 22,
        40, 60, 64, 65, 66, 92

Iowa Program centered in, 15
Mabie as head, 29
Mabie period ends, 160
Merry and scientific program in, 9
Program degrees in, 123
Program migrating into, 90
Phonology, phonetics, laboratory
    courses in, 10
Psychology, Iowa Program, and, 6
Public Speaking unit of, 9
scientific orientation in, 29-30
sponsor of Program, with others,
    116, 117
takes Speech half of Psychology and
    Speech Clinic, 117
Speech and Hearing Center, Wendell
    Johnson
    see Wendell Johnson Speech and
        Hearing Center
Speech and hearing disorders
    and communication, 66
    and speech correction, 25-26
    discovered in fundamentals course
        sections, 11, 12, 22, 40, 60, 64,
        65, 66, 92
    first doctoral-level training in, 14
    found in WPA survey, 93
    in East Hall clinic, 65
    initial research thrust in, 21
    in schools, 78-79
        see also hearing testing
            Iowa Program in Speech
                Pathology
            organic speech and hearing
                disorders
            speech pathology
            stuttering
            (in preceding index) Mabie,
                Merry
Speech and Hearing Mobile Clinic,
    50-51
Speech breathing, 169
Speech Clinic
    and Head Start, 194
    and laboratory, 30-31
    and migrant workers, 194
    and Regional Educational Services
        Administration, 194
    and sectioned fundamentals class,
        22
    as one with Psychological Clinic, 88
    at Veterans Administration

Hospital, 181-182
  Barrows' work in, 21
  caseload of, 123, 193-194
  catalogue listing of, 130
  committee for, 22-23
  confusing titles of, 60, 70-71
  forerunner of, 65-66
  foreshadowed, 11-12
  listed in catalogue, 74
  Petersen as, 45-46
  reorganization of, 158, 185-186
  separated from Psychological Clinic,
    117
  see also Services
Speech correction
  and Hawk, 44
  and Ogdahl, 51
  and Sherman, 78-79
  early history of, 73
  grouping in catalogue list, 25-26
  in schools, 78-79, 93, 155, 166-167,
    173, 193
  in state institutions, 142-144
  Powers and Chicago division of, 43
  training for, 79
  WPA school survey of need for, 93
Speech pathologist(s)
  as new term, 25
  early, 40-51
  first, 20
  out of fundamentals course staff,
    11-12
Speech pathology
  as major discipline, 49
  as new term, 25
  as parent of audiology, 107-108
  first 25 years of, 3
  clinical psychology, Psychopathic
    Hospital, and, 3
  gains national organization (ASHA),
    26-27
  in East Hall, 65
  maturing of, 86
  plea for major in, 123
  separated from general speech, 29
  see also Iowa Program in Speech
    Pathology and Audiology,
  Speech Pathology and Audiology,
  Speech Pathology and Audiology,
    Department of
Speech pathology and audiology
  Council created for, 127-129

given catalogue listing, 130-131
  granted department status, 154
  grows nationally, 165-166
  two disciplines joined in, 107-108
Speech Pathology and Audiology,
  Department of,
  and Hospital School, 180
  and Psychology, 180
  and Psychology and Speech, 65
  created in Curtis period, 154,
    161-162
  projection to 1978 for, 203-205
  purposes of, 204
  reports of, 166-170, 172-174,
    175-177, 178-179, 181-182,
    189-190, 195, 203-205
  Seashore and, 65
Speech Pathology Laboratory
  basic to Iowa Program, 30-31
  built by Travis and Hunter, 33-36
  called Phonetics and Speech
    Laboratory, 130
  in Psychopathic Hospital, 65
  moved to East Hall, 70
  space problems of and Curtis
    request, 125-126
  Smith contact with, 50
  see also Speech science
Speech Pathology and Audiology
  Laboratory
  see Phonetics and Speech
    Laboratory
Speech science
  and computer, 130
  and Curtis laboratory, 130
  beginnings, 9-12
  Curtis and, 103-104
  early listings in, 73
  Fairbanks and, 42-43
  growth in NRC years, 29-30
  in Curtis period, 135, 154, 155, 203,
    205
  Lynch and, 49
  Merry degree and program in, 21
  new undergraduate major in, 183,
    189-190
  see also Phonetics and Speech
    Laboratory,
      Speech and Hearing Science,
      Speech Pathology
        Laboratory
Speech sounds and graphic
  representation, 11

Speech therapy
    early, 71
    in state institutions, 142-144
    see also Curriculum,
            Psychological and Speech
                Clinic
            Psychological Clinic,
            Speech Clinic,
            Speech Correction
Spirometer, 180
Student counseling office as offspring,
    105
Stuttering
    adaptation and consistency in, 76
    and "cure," 20
    and Demosthenes Club, 92-93
    and early clinical work, 88
    and General Semantics, 105-106,
        114
    and handedness, 33, 36, 50, 61-62
    and Johnson Thesis, 63
    and shock, 27-28
    and speechlessness, 42
    and sporadic institutions, 3
    and two reunions, 139-140
    avoidance theory of, 76
    bounce technique in, 77-78
    bulk of research in, 97
    capital of world for, 113
    dominance theory of, 16, 33, 55, 61,
        62, 63
    early studies of in theses, 8, 20, 40,
        49, 50, 63-64
    emphasized by Johnson, 114
    loci of, 94
    measuring severity of, 47
    moment of, 75-76, 94
    pioneer research in, 20
    pistol and study of, 27-28
    prediction in, 76
    program in Curtis period, 155, 169,
        203
    psychosocial approach to, 133-135
    rejection of neurological approach,
        78
    theory, early, 75-78
    therapy for, 71, 72
    voluntary, 62, 78
Stutterer(s)
    and scholars, 44-45
    as guinea pig, 62
    as research subjects, 36-37
    as white rat, 61-62
    attracted by Travis work, 41-42
    in glib society, 64
Summer Clinic
    see Residential Clinic

Tape recorder and Johnson, 140-141
Templin-Darley Tests, 169-170
Theories as Iowa hallmark, 63
Timbre, 47
Tone and cadaver, 61
Tonoscope, 4
Tuning forks, 2, 67

University Bulletin and Psychology
    (diagram), 20
University Hospital and clinical
    psychology, 87
University Hospital School and
    Strother, 108-109

Vacuum tube in early research, 36
Velopharyngeal valving studies, 169
Voice, 10, 11, 18, 27, 66
    and articulation, 22, 88, 102, 120,
        156
    and phonetics
        Fairbanks and, 42
        pioneering in science of, 21, 22
        see also Speech science
    disorders, 203
    quality, 136
    science, 26

Wendell Johnson Speech and Hearing
    Center (photo 206)
    application for federal funds for,
        182
    contract let for, 182, 187
    dedication of, 199-202
    Department's move into, 192
    federal grants for, 187
    in Curtis period, 154, 159
    Johnson plaque in, 206
    recommendation for, 179
    state funds voted for, 180-181
    summer clinic moved to, 187
Wood for winter warmth, 4
Workshops, 146
WPA school survey in speech and
    hearing, 93
World War II
    and audiology, 107-108
    and Iowa Program group, 100-101

and returning veterans, 115
maturing of audiology, speech
    pathology, clinical psychology
    during, 86-87

problems generated by, 86, 87, 88,
    96
reflected in 1941-1942 catalogue,
    95-96